Staying Strong

A Senior's Guide to a More Active and Independent Life

Edited by Lorie A. Schleck, MA, PT

Fairview Press
Minneapolis, Minnesota

Published by Fairview Press, 2450 Riverside Avenue, Minneapolis, MN 55454.

Cataloging-in-Publication Data
Staying strong : a senior's guide to a more active and independent life / edited by Lorie Schleck ; [photography by Anna Esser].
     p. cm.
  ISBN 1-57749-097-5 (pbk. : alk. paper)
    1. Physical fitness for the aged. 2. Exercise for the aged.
  I. Title: Senior's guide to a more active and independent life.
  II. Schleck, Lorie.

GV447 .S82 2000
613.7'0446--dc21   00-057833

First Printing: November 2000

Printed in the United States of America
04 03 02 01 00   7 6 5 4 3 2 1

Photographs: Anna Esser
Interior: Spring Type and Design
Cover: *Cover design by Laurie Ingram Duren*™

We'd like to thank our models: Mabel Erickson, Doloris Haakenson, Helmer Hanka, Lillian Lazenberry, James Lincoln, Ruth Passage, Cookie Sarenpa, and James Small.

For a free current catalog of Fairview Press titles, please call toll-free 1-800-544-8207 or visit our web site at *www.fairviewpress.org*.

To Jim, my husband and best friend.

Contents

1

Strength Training for Older Adults

Lorie A. Schleck, MA, PT

A recent study of older Americans found that seven out of ten women over age 70 are unable to lift 10 pounds. Yes, that's right. Seven out of ten older women cannot lift even 10 pounds! And this is not just a "female" problem. Seven out of twenty men over age 70 are just as frail. Think of the normal, everyday activities that become difficult if not impossible when you can't lift 10 pounds of weight: grocery shopping, vacuuming, working in the yard, doing the laundry, carrying a suitcase or heavy purse, holding a child, opening containers, getting in and out of a bathtub or deep chair, opening a window, moving pots and pans, setting the table, watering plants, walking a dog, shoveling snow, changing bedding. The list could go on and on. What happens when you can't do these activities by yourself? You depend on others to do them for you. And, in some cases, you lose the pleasures and benefits of these activities altogether.

All of us want to remain as active and independent as possible for as long as we can. All of us want to maintain a high quality of life as we age. The question is, can we do it, and if so, how?

Dorothy is a 75-year-old retired school teacher who maintains an active social life. She is very involved at her church and loves to travel, having taken two longs trips to Africa in the last few years. Except for a recent hip replacement, Dorothy has no major or chronic health concerns. She regularly visits nursing homes, cheering the occupants with her positive outlook and exuberant energy. Aerobic exercise and strength training are a routine part of Dorothy's week.

Why do some people, like Dorothy, maintain good health and an active lifestyle well into retirement, while many others experience ill health and loss of independence?

In the last decade we have learned that healthy aging is not simply a matter of fate or good genetics. Abundant scientific evidence has shown that maintaining muscular strength plays an important role in successful aging. Because Dorothy chooses to make strength training a part of her regular routine, she enjoys a healthy, vibrant lifestyle that has taken her halfway around the world.

WHAT IS STRENGTH TRAINING?

Mention strength training and a vision of youthful bodies lifting big barbells comes to mind. Few people associate strength training with older adults. But with some minor modifications, biceps curls and leg extensions are every bit as appropriate for those of us in our sixth, seventh, or even eighth and ninth decade of life. And the health benefits are tremendous.

The concept is simple: Strength training is any activity that moves a body part against resistance. Resistance may be isometric (when you tighten a muscle and hold it for several seconds), or it might involve a small weight, a household object, or an exercise band (a 3- or 4-foot elastic band designed for exercise).

Strength training does not require a gym or membership in a health club. It need not involve expensive or heavy equipment. If we know a few simple principles and learn some basic exercises, we can do strength training at home, at the park, or with a group of friends.

WHY STRENGTH TRAIN?

Few older adults exercise to look good in a swimsuit. For most of us, strength training is critical to maintaining our health and our independence. The benefits of strength training are considerable—and these benefits become evident in a very short time.

Bigger, Stronger Muscles

When we reach middle age, we begin to lose muscle mass. Our muscles literally begin to shrink and weaken. This is a natural process that medical professionals call *sarcopenia*. Once we hit age 70, our muscle loss accelerates. We may find it difficult to go up and down the stairs. A grocery bag or laundry basket may become too heavy. We might feel wobbly when walking across the room.

Weakness, difficulty with everyday activities, frail arms and legs—these are *not* the inevitable results of age. When it comes to aging muscles, an old saying applies: "Use it or lose it."

In the absence of major health problems, regular strength training leads to noticeably stronger muscles in only six to eight weeks, no matter what your age. One study of strength training in older men found that participants doubled the strength of their quadriceps after just three months. The quadriceps muscle, which runs along the front of the thigh, is critical for going up and down stairs and rising from a chair or toilet. To maintain (or regain) a basic level of independence, it is crucial to keep this muscle strong.

Hilmer is a 65-year-old retired high school principal and basketball coach. Although he walks for thirty minutes, three or four times each week, he has recently noticed little changes in his physical abilities. Climbing the stairs requires greater effort. An hour of gardening leaves him sore and stiff the next day. It has become difficult to lift a golf bag. At his next physical, Hilmer discusses his concerns with his physician. The doctor commends Hilmer for walking regularly, but he recommends a simple exercise program to strengthen some important muscles.

Hilmer follows his doctor's recommendation. After six weeks he notices that simple daily tasks, like lifting a pan from the oven and pushing the mower across the lawn, are getting easier. Now, as he continues his strengthening exercises twice a week, Hilmer is lifting his golf bag as easily as he did fifteen years ago.

Stronger Bones

Strength training is one of the most important steps we can take to prevent osteoporosis and subsequent fractures. Osteoporosis, or loss of bone density, is a major health concern for older adults, particularly women. When bones lose density, they become weaker, making them more susceptible to fractures. Broken bones are not only painful, they can be life threatening as well.

Although osteoporosis cannot be cured, it can be prevented. Over the last decade, research has shown that regular strength training can help us strengthen our bones and avoid this potentially debilitating disease. And for those of us who already have osteoporosis, strength training can help us maintain or rebuild bone mass in our spine, hips, and wrists—the areas most susceptible to fracture.

Improved Balance

As we age, we may begin to feel wobbly or off-balance, a condition that could lead to falls and serious injury. For some of us, walking, showering, even bending over to pick up a book may cause us to lose our balance.

Balance is a complex process involving muscles, nerves, and the vestibular system (an important part of the inner ear). Balance problems are often a sign of muscle weakness—as we exercise and rebuild our muscle strength, our balance generally improves. Better balance reduces our chances of falling and makes simple daily tasks, like walking and showering, safer.

Fewer Falls

Falls are one of the most serious and common medical problems suffered by older adults. Every year, about one-third of people over 65 experience a fall. Falls cause bruises, fractures, and other injuries. And, once we have suffered a fall, we often develop a fear of falling that prevents us from participating in our normal activities.

Strong muscles decrease our chances of falling. If a fall does occur, strong muscles help protect our bones, making us less likely to experience a fracture or other serious injury.

Daily Tasks Are Easier

Most of us strength train because we want to improve our "functional strength." Functional strength is the amount of strength we need to accomplish our daily tasks. For example, if the washing machine is in the basement, we need to be strong enough to carry a load of laundry up and down the stairs. When grocery shopping, we must be strong enough to carry the groceries into the house from the car.

One study found that people between 75 and 80 years of age who led sedentary lives used more than half their muscular strength just to take a shower. This is not an inevitable sign of age—this is a sign of muscle weakness. Regular strength training will prevent or reverse this muscle loss, giving us the strength we need in our daily lives.

Improved Mobility

Crossing the street before the light changes, climbing the stairs to our third-floor apartment, walking to the mailbox without running out of breath—when modest goals like these become difficult, they jeopardize our independence.

Through strength training, we can improve our walking speed as well as our ability to climb stairs. In fact, strength training allows many of us to continue living in our homes long after our peers have moved to assisted living facilities.

Increased Activity Level

For many of us, the saying: "My get-up-and-go, got up and went" is a little too familiar. Feeling tired and weak, we might limit ourselves to sedentary activities, like watching television or reading on the couch. But when we begin strength training, we are surprised to find that we feel like doing more. We rediscover our "get-up-and-go."

In one study, a group of nursing home residents began regular strength-training sessions. They quickly started feeling stronger and doing more. In fact, their spontaneous physical activity increased by almost 30 percent. They began to prefer walking over sitting, and moving over being still.

Better Weight Control

Strength training, especially when combined with aerobic exercise, is a surefire way to control body weight. Why? Because muscle burns calories and fat. The more muscle we have, the more calories we burn.

But left to its own devices, the body loses about a half pound of muscle every year after age 30. If we don't keep ourselves strong, we gain weight with each passing year.

If your goal is to lose weight or maintain your figure, strength training can help in two ways. First, your body burns calories and fat while you exercise. Second, when your muscles are strong and well-toned, your metabolism increases, causing your body to burn even more calories and fat all day long.

You can think of metabolism as how your body burns fuel (fat and calories) during the day. You burn fuel whenever you move, but also when you're at rest. (Imagine an idling car engine—even when it isn't moving, it needs fuel to keep running.) As your muscles become stronger, your body must burn more fuel. Even if your strength-training sessions last only thirty minutes every other day, your metabolism can be elevated throughout the whole day, every day. You can even burn more calories in your sleep!

But remember, muscle weighs more than fat. This means that you may lose inches, but not necessarily pounds. As the fat melts away, it is replaced with strong, toned muscles, so the news from the bathroom scale may not seem encouraging. Do not despair. You will likely lose inches in critical places, like the waist and hips. You will look thinner and feel better, even if you don't lose much weight. Trust how you feel and look—don't measure your success with the bathroom scale.

When George received a notice for his forty-year class reunion, he decided that the tire around his waist and those few—well, more than a few—extra pounds had to go. George checked with his doctor and started a strength-training program. But as he stepped on the scale each week, the pounds weren't dropping off as he had expected. Just when he started to get frustrated, he began to hear compliments from his friends and family: "George, you're looking good." "Are you losing weight, George?"

George went to his class reunion feeling good about his appearance. He had dropped several inches around the waist, even though he had shed only a few pounds.

COMMONLY ASKED QUESTIONS

This sounds too good to be true. Why haven't I heard it before?

Gerontology, or the study of aging, is a relatively new science. For a time, gerontology focused on disease and declining health—conditions associated with aging. But in the last decade or so, science has begun to focus on aging healthily. Since then, research has shown that lifestyle choices play a critical role in determining our health, no matter what our age.

Strength training is one of the most important choices we can make. In fact, so much evidence has accumulated to support the link between good strength and good health that the American College of Sports Medicine recently revised its exercise recommendations for the first time in over a decade. They now recommend that every adult participate in a regular strength-training program.

Is strength training safe?

Strength training is safe for almost everyone. But, as with any exercise program, it's important to check with your doctor before you begin. If you take certain medications or suffer from a specific medical condition, strength training may cause undesirable—or even dangerous—symptoms.

If you perform your exercises correctly, the risk of injury is minimal. The most common reason for injury, regardless of a person's age, is trying to progress too quickly. The next chapter outlines some simple safety tips and other important information—be sure to review this before beginning your strength-training program.

Is strength training all I need to do?

Strength training is just one part of a healthy lifestyle. You're probably familiar with the other parts: good nutrition, aerobic exercise (such as walking), and stretching exercises. Among people aged 65 to 74, two-thirds of women and three-fourths of men participate in some type of regular physical activity. But only 7 percent of men and 3 percent of women participate in a regular strength-training program. It's time to get the word out: As older adults, we need strength training to maintain (or regain) our health.

How do I get started?

With such compelling evidence supporting the link between regular strength training and good health, it's time to get started. The next chapter outlines some simple, but important, guidelines for a safe and effective strength-training program.

Lorie A. Schleck is a physical therapist at Fairview Rehabilitation Services. She received her BS degree in physical therapy from the University of Minnesota and her MA degree in counseling psychology from St. Mary's University of Minnesota. Lorie and her husband, Jim, have a son, Ben, and a daughter, Kara.

2

Before You Get Started

Mike Muffenbier, MPT, SCS, CSCS
Lorie A. Schleck, MA, PT

The facts are in: Strength training is one of the most important lifestyle choices we can make, especially if we're over age 50. In the following chapters, you will find a number of strength-training programs designed to help you reach specific goals. But before you jump in, you'll need to consider some cautions and guidelines that will make your strengthening program safer and more effective.

WHEN TO TAKE PRECAUTIONS

First, anytime you make a significant change in your normal health routine—such as starting a strengthening program—discuss it with your doctor. He or she can alert you to any health conditions or medications that might make strength training difficult or unsafe.

If you have an **orthopedic injury** or **chronic joint or back problems,** you may need to modify the exercises. Your physician, or perhaps a physical therapist, will be able to advise you.

Individuals with **high blood pressure (hypertension)** should exercise with caution, because blood pressure may rise during strength training. If your blood pressure is well-controlled AND your doctor has given permission, you should be able to strength train safely. However, you must use a low level of resistance, and you must always remain conscious of your breathing. Do not hold your breath while exercising.

If you have been diagnosed with **osteoporosis,** you must be careful not to stress certain areas of your body. The osteoporosis program in chapter 5 will allow you to strength train with very little risk of injury; however, you should check with your doctor before starting this program. And to make sure you are doing the exercises correctly, you may want to do your first few sessions under the care of a physical therapist.

Heart disease, too, deserves special consideration. Depending on the type and severity of your heart disease, you may need to take precautions and be alert to dangerous symptoms. Consult your doctor before beginning any kind of exercise program.

If you suffer from **arthritis,** do not exercise during periods of active pain and inflammation. Do your exercises slowly and gently, and only during periods of minimal pain. Again, check with your doctor before starting a strength-training program.

**Medical Conditions
Warranting Special Caution**
- Orthopedic injury
- Chronic joint or back pain
- High blood pressure
- Osteoporosis
- Heart Disease
- Arthritis

This book contains eight strength-training programs. The guide on pages 13 and 14 will help you decide which program is right for you.

Selecting a Strength-Training Program

Reason/ Condition	General	Osteoporosis Prevention	Osteoporosis	Balance	Golf	Pool	Chair	Bed	Comments
Morning Stiffness								x	Begin your day with the Bed program. If able, do another program later in the day 2 to 3 times/week.
Recent Joint Replacement	x					x			Follow the instructions given by your doctor or physical therapist.
Recent Broken Hip	x					x		x	Begin with Bed program, then progress to the Pool or to General Strength Training.
Balance Problems				x		x	x		
Recent Heart Attack	x								Follow your doctor's instructions. Upper body exercises are more taxing on the heart, so be conservative with these.
Recent Surgery	x					x			Avoid exercises that cause pain.
Arthritis						x	x	x	Use the Bed program to alleviate morning stiffness. A warm pool works best for the Pool program.
Chronic Back Pain	x					x			Avoid exercises that increase pain.
Muscle/Joint Problems	x					x			Avoid exercises that increase pain.
Foot Problems						x	x		

Reason/ Condition	General	Osteoporosis Prevention	Osteoporosis	Balance	Golf	Pool	Chair	Bed	Comments
Diabetes	x						x		General Strength Training builds strength and increases circulation. If you have a foot or leg problem, try the Chair program.
Lung Disease	x								Take longer rests if needed. If shortness of breath occurs, stop immediately.
Post-Menopausal		x							
Osteoporosis			x						
Golf Player					x				
Goal of Weight Loss	x								Work up to three sets of 10 to 15 repetitions.
Goal of Increased Fitness	x								
Confined to Wheelchair							x		
Use a Walker or Cane	x						x		If able, do the General Strength Training program while holding on to a sturdy chair. If too unsteady, use the Chair program.
Recent Illness	x						x	x	If you are very weak, start with the Bed program, progress to the Chair, then to General Strength Training.

GETTING STARTED

As we've said before, you won't need any heavy equipment or fancy clothes for strength training. In fact, you'll find most of the equipment around your house—a towel, a belt, a sturdy chair. (Be sure to select a chair that won't tip over when you lean on it. For seated exercises, you will need a chair with armrests.)

Some exercises require a resistance band—a 3- or 4-foot elastic band that provides resistance when stretched. Your muscles will work against this resistance. Thera-Band® is a favorite brand of resistance band. Thera-Band exercise bands are very inexpensive, and they are color coded according to the amount of resistance they offer. In this book, we refer only to the color system used by Thera-Band. Other bands use different colors, so check with the manufacturer of the brand you choose. (NOTE: Thera-Band produces both latex and latex-free exercise bands. If you think you might be allergic to latex, be sure to buy the latex-free bands, which are clearly marked with the words "latex free.") Thera-Band exercise bands are available at most sporting goods stores, or you can order them by calling 1-800-321-2135.

Finally, you'll need to select comfortable clothes for exercising. Wear loose-fitting, nonbinding clothes that allow you to move without restriction. You'll also need a pair of sturdy athletic shoes with plenty of arch support. Walking shoes, running shoes, or tennis shoes should provide enough stability.

A COMPLETE FITNESS PROGRAM

A complete fitness program consists of four parts: aerobic exercise, warm-up, strength training, and stretching exercises. The programs in this book provide all but the aerobic exercise. You will have to do aerobic exercises on your own.

Aerobic Exercise

Aerobic exercises—such as walking, biking, swimming, and cross-country skiing—are activities that specifically improve cardiovascular fitness. Medical experts recommend at least thirty minutes of aerobic exercise three or more times each week.

For more information on aerobic exercise, talk to your doctor, visit your local health club, or browse the fitness section in your nearest bookstore.

Warm-up

Before doing any kind of exercise, your body needs to warm up. Without an adequate warm-up, strength training may be painful and difficult—and you'll be more likely to injure yourself.

You will find a complete warm-up at the start of each strength-training program in this book. The purpose of the warm-up is to get your heart beating a little harder and the blood pumping a little faster so your muscles are ready to work.

A warm-up generally involves four or five minutes of simple movements with your arms and legs, but any fairly vigorous activity will do. Walking your dog or mowing the lawn is an excellent warm-up for strength training.

Strength Training

Muscles get stronger when they work against resistance, such as an exercise band. Unless your doctor says otherwise, resistance should be progressive—as your strength increases, you'll need to add more resistance by using the next level of exercise band.

You will do repetitions, or reps, of all the exercises in your program. For each exercise, you will move from starting position, through the range of motion, and back to the starting position—this is one rep.

Once you have chosen an appropriate strength-training program, practice doing 10 reps of each exercise without a resistance band. This will give your joints and muscles time to adjust to the movements. It will also help you determine your comfortable range of motion for each exercise.

When you feel ready to work with a Thera-Band exercise band, begin with the yellow color—the least resistance—and do 10 reps of each exercise. Some muscles may be stronger than others, so if certain exercises seem too easy, you may add more resistance during those exercises.

The more a band is stretched, the more resistance it provides. No matter what color band you're using, try to create the same amount of "stretch" each time you work out.

Our strengthening program—which is based on the color system used by Thera-Band—consists of six levels. At Level I, you will do 10 reps of each exercise using a yellow band. When 10 reps become easy, you will progress to 12 reps, and then to 15. When 15 reps become easy, it's time to progress to Level II, the red band. Because the red band provides more resistance, you will drop back down to 10 reps, then you'll build up to 12, and then to 15. You will continue this pattern through each level until you reach your desired level of strength. (Remember, this is the color system used by Thera-Band. Different manufacturers will use different color systems.)

Levels of Strength Training
Using Thera-Band Exercise Bands

No Band	I (Yellow) light	II (Red) medium	III (Green) heavy	IV (Blue) extra heavy	V (Black) special heavy	VI (Silver) super heavy
10 reps (first few sessions)	10 reps	10 reps	10 reps	10 reps	10 reps	10 reps
	12 reps	12 reps	12 reps	12 reps	12 reps	12 reps
	15 reps	15 reps	15 reps	15 reps	15 reps	15 reps

Progression Plan

Do not progress too quickly. Ten reps with any band may be difficult at first, but each session will get a little easier. Stay with 10 reps until you can finish each exercise without difficulty. This may take two or three sessions; it may take a dozen or more.

You might move quickly through the first level or two, but progress will slow as resistance increases. Listen to your body— you'll know when you're ready to go to the next level. The number-one cause of injury is trying to progress too fast. Give your body time to adjust to the demands of strength training. The older you are, the more time you'll need to adjust.

Frequency

To see results, you'll need to strength train two or three times a week; however, your body needs forty-eight hours of rest between sessions. This means that you shouldn't strength train two days in a row. On days when you're not strength training, you may want to do aerobic or stretching exercises.

Advancing

No strength-training program will make you stronger and stronger indefinitely. You will occasionally reach a plateau, or a pause in the progression of your program. For example, you might sail through Level I, needing only three sessions at 10, 12, and 15 reps. But when you get to Level II, you may need many more sessions at 10 reps before you can advance to 12 reps. Be patient with yourself; these plateaus are normal. In time, the exercises will get easier, and your body will be ready to move on.

Maintenance

Whether your goal is to keep up with daily chores or play eighteen holes of golf several times a week, you will likely build the strength you need for your lifestyle. At that point, you will begin the maintenance phase of your program.

Once you reach your desired level of strength, do not advance to the next level; simply continue at the current level and repeat your program two or three times a week. If you stop, you will begin to lose the strength you have worked so hard to build.

When 75-year-old Ruth realized that common activities—like climbing stairs and rising from the toilet—were becoming difficult, her doctor recommended a strength-training program. Always enthusiastic, Ruth quickly advanced through Level I and most of Level II. But for several weeks, she just couldn't advance to Level III.

Feeling somewhat discouraged, Ruth remembered her doctor's advice: "At some point, you will hit a plateau. It may take weeks, but if you keep exercising, you'll get to the next level." Ruth kept at it, and soon she was advancing through Level III.

By then, Ruth realized that her daily tasks had become easier. She had reached her goal. Today, Ruth continues to strength train at Level III, two or three times a week, in order to maintain her muscle strength.

Chances are, your progress will look different from Ruth's. (For a diagram of Ruth's progress, see the following page.) Your program might move more slowly or more quickly. You may have many more plateaus—or none at all. Perhaps your goal is to run the local marathon, so you need to reach a higher level of strength. Remember, strength training varies from person to person. Always listen to your body. Know your goals, and progress only when you are ready.

Ruth's Progress

	Week 1-5	Week 6-10	Week 11-13	Week 14-20
Level III: Green				
15 reps				• • • • • • •
				Maintenance Phase
12 reps			•	
10 reps			•	
Level II: Red				
15 reps		• • • • •		
		Plateau Phase		
12 reps		•		
10 reps		•		
Level I: Yellow				
15 reps	•			
12 reps	•			
10 reps	•			
No band				
10 reps	•			

Week 1 2 3 4 5 6 7 8 9 10 11 12 13 14 15 16 17 18 19 20

Stretching Exercises

Many people associate aging with accumulating aches and pains. As we grow older, our muscles tend to become tighter and our joints lose mobility. This makes it difficult—and sometimes painful—to accomplish simple tasks, like reaching overhead to get a plate from the top shelf or reaching across our body to fasten our seat belt.

The cure for muscle tightness is simple: regular stretching exercises. Studies show that sore muscles and stiff joints are often related to loss of flexibility. Stretching loosens up those muscles and joints, making everyday movements easier and less painful.

Here's another reason to stretch: Strength training causes muscles to contract, or shorten. In time, this can lead to muscle tightness. But just as strength training can cause muscle shortening, stretching exercises will aid muscle lengthening.

Each strength-training program in this book includes essential stretching exercises designed to increase flexibility in key areas (easing the aches and pains associated with age), and to restore normal muscle length after strength training. Do these stretches every time you complete a strength-training session.

TECHNIQUES

The strength-training programs in this book are very simple—they do not involve fancy equipment or advanced techniques—but there are important considerations you'll want to keep in mind.

Breathing

Many strength-training programs recommend a pattern of breathing where you inhale as you move against resistance and exhale as you return to the starting position. Because the programs in this book involve steady, slow movements, this breathing technique will not work.

During strength training, your breathing should be relaxed and natural. Keep your mouth open so you can breathe freely. Do not take deep breaths. It is critical that you NEVER, EVER HOLD YOUR BREATH: Holding your breath while strength training can be dangerous, so make a conscious effort to breathe normally. If you find yourself short of breath, you are working too hard. Stop at once.

Form

Most strength-training exercises are done either seated or standing. Throughout each exercise, it's important to maintain proper body alignment.

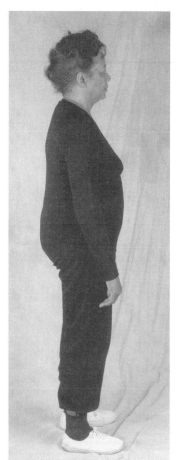

For standing exercises, you should stand tall and straight. Be careful not to thrust your head forward or bend at the waist.

For seated exercises, sit up tall with both feet planted firmly on the floor. You may want to use a rolled-up towel to support your lower back.

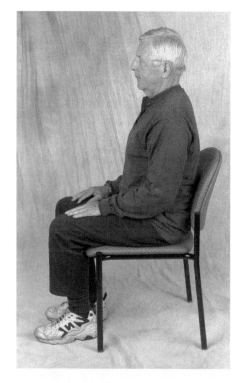

If you have a hard time maintaining proper body alignment, you are probably working too hard. Decrease the resistance and try again. If you are still struggling, try the exercise without the exercise band, and add resistance only when you can maintain proper body alignment.

Pace

Pace describes the rate at which your body moves while exercising. Every movement should be slow, smooth, and deliberate. Move into the resistance to a slow count of 2, then return to the starting position to a slow count of 4. Remember:
- Never jerk on the resistance band.
- Do not rock your body.
- Never move explosively.

A slow, smooth pace will make your strength training safer and more productive.

Rest

If you are doing several sets of a given exercise, take a short rest between sets. After completing one set of 10 to 15 repetitions, wait thirty seconds before beginning another set. This gives your muscles time to replenish some of the energy they have just used up.

Range of Motion

Do your exercises in a PAIN-FREE range of motion. If any of your movements are limited for any reason, you may need to modify certain exercises. For example, if an exercise requires you to sit in a chair and extend your leg, straighten the leg only as far as you can without causing pain.

GOALS

Strength training is different from bodybuilding. The goal of bodybuilding is to build big muscles for show. The goal of strength training is to build stronger muscles—whether for an independent lifestyle, for recreation, or for improved athletic performance.

No matter what your goals are, avoid giving yourself a deadline: "I want to be strong enough to carry a bag of leaves to the curb in six weeks" or "I want to lift my golf bag in and out of my trunk in eight weeks." When you add time constraints, you're more likely to overdo it. Also, some people progress faster than others. A realistic goal for one person might not be realistic for another. But one thing is for sure: If you follow the program guidelines, you will get stronger. Be patient and give your body the time it needs to advance.

Functional strength is the core goal of a strengthening program. Recreational and athletic strength can be added to this primary goal.

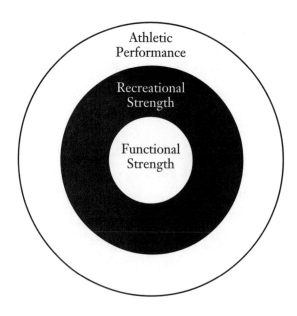

Goal #1: Functional Strength

Every adult over age 50 needs a basic level of strength in the major muscle groups. We must be strong enough to carry a bag of garbage to the garage and to lift it into the garbage can. Or to carry a load of laundry to the washing machine. Or to lift ourselves out of our favorite chair at the end of the ball game. This is called functional strength—the level of strength we need to perform our daily tasks.

Is your primary goal to maintain your health and independence? Perhaps daily tasks are becoming more difficult:

- carrying a bag full of leaves to the curb.
- getting in and out of the bathtub easily.
- carrying a pot of coffee.
- climbing up and down the stairs without becoming tired.
- rising from the toilet without support or assistance.

If functional strength is your goal, strength training will help you build muscle and complete your daily tasks with ease. But don't quit the program! To maintain your strength, you'll need to continue strength training on a regular basis. Otherwise, you will lose the muscle strength you have worked so hard to build.

Goal #2: Recreational Strength

Beyond a need for functional strength, many of us have recreational goals. If we expect to enjoy our activities for many years to come, our muscles must be up to the task. A daily walk, several sets of tennis, eighteen holes of golf, or an occupation that involves significant physical effort—all demand a certain amount of strength. If we plan to continue an active lifestyle, strength training is the key.

If your goals are recreational, your strength training must progress farther because you need greater strength. Again, consider your specific goals. You may want to:

- easily lift your golf bag in and out of the trunk of your car.
- walk up the hill near your house without having to rest.
- jog 3 miles in thirty-five minutes.

Once you have met your goals, begin the maintenance phase of your program. You must continue strength training or your muscle strength will decrease.

If you want a more intense workout, you might try two or even three sets of repetitions for each exercise. But use caution: More sets mean you're more likely to overdo it. As a general rule, most people over age fifty need only one set of repetitions. Two or three sets are only recommended for people who are very active and whose goals require a significant amount of strength.

Goal #3: Improved Athletic Performance

Some of us are involved in athletics, where improved performance is the primary objective. If the goal is to become a scratch golfer or train for the local race, strength training needs to be more focused and intense. Perhaps your goal is to:
- better your time in the 5-kilometer race by thirty seconds.
- drive the golf ball 10 yards farther off the tee.
- improve your tennis game by adding power to your forehand and backhand, so you can move up in club rankings.

Athletic goals require the greatest amount of fitness and strength. For a more intense workout, you may need to do two or three sets of repetitions for each exercise. Again, don't quit the program once you have reached your goals. You will need to continue regular strength training to maintain your desired level of strength.

WHAT TO EXPECT

You may wonder, will strength training hurt? Will I get big muscles? How will I know if I'm doing something wrong? When will I feel stronger?

Strength training takes some effort. The exercises should leave you tired, but never exhausted. If you are completely fatigued, you're overdoing it—take a few days off and resume your program at a lower intensity (decrease the resistance or the number of repetitions, or both). Strength-training exercises should not cause pain. If you experience pain, stop immediately.

Good Soreness versus Bad Pain

You will likely experience some muscle soreness at first. This typically occurs a day or two after starting your program, and it can last one week. Soreness may return whenever you increase the intensity of your workout. This soreness is normal and to be expected. If you're not sure whether your soreness is good or bad, consider the location, onset, and type:

	Good Soreness	**Bad Pain**
Location	Muscle	Bone or joint
Onset	1–2 days after starting exercise (or after increasing exercise intensity)	During exercise
Type	Vague, diffuse	Sharp, acute

If you feel sore, wait until the soreness has diminished before exercising again.

Every now and then, you will miss several strength-training sessions in a row. A vacation in the Bahamas or a bout with the flu, for example, may force you to take time off. When you return to your program, decrease the intensity of your workout: Try fewer repetitions or a less-resistant exercise band (or both). Then, gradually build back up to an appropriate level. The more sessions you miss, the less intense your workout should be. This will minimize your muscle soreness after you resume exercising.

Body Changes

Don't expect to see immediate changes in your body—it will take several sessions before you notice a difference in strength and endurance. In the first four to six weeks, your muscles and nerves are learning to work more efficiently. Muscle size and shape only begin to change after six to eight weeks of consistent strength training. Only then will you see real changes in muscle strength. At that point, you may notice firmer, more toned muscles.

TIME TO GET STARTED

Now that you know what to expect, it's time to start exercising. The following chapters outline specific programs designed to meet your particular needs. You can decide which program is right for you. No matter which one you choose, remember this cardinal rule: **Listen to your body**.

Mike Muffenbier is a physical therapist with Fairview Rehabilitation Services, where he works in sports medicine. A board-certified specialist in sports physical therapy, Mike is also a certified strength and conditioning specialist. He teaches shoulder and knee rehabilitation, along with exercise program design, to professionals throughout the country. Mike and his wife, Michelle, have two daughters, Ali and Bailey.

Lorie A. Schleck is a physical therapist at Fairview Rehabilitation Services. She received her BS degree in physical therapy from the University of Minnesota and her MA degree in counseling psychology from St. Mary's University of Minnesota. Lorie and her husband, Jim, have a son, Ben, and a daughter, Kara.

3

General Strength Training

Kecia E. Sell, MS, PT, ATC/R
Lorie A. Schleck, MA, PT

This program takes about 30 minutes.
Do it 2 to 3 times each week.
A 48-hour break is recommended between each session.

EQUIPMENT NEEDED:
   Stable, heavy chair that will not tip over
   Chair or stool
   Length of resistance band (3 to 4 feet)
   Loop of resistance band

General Strength Training is appropriate for anyone who wants to improve the strength of key muscle groups for overall health. It is also designed to make many daily tasks, such as yard work and housework, easier.

THE PROGRAM

General Strength Training consists of a warm-up session, strengthening exercises, and warm-down stretching exercises. You may want to meet with a physical therapist or other health-care professional before beginning this program. A trained professional can help make sure you are exercising properly.

Exercise Guidelines
- Wear comfortable, nonbinding clothing.
- Maintain proper body alignment:
  - For standing exercises, stand tall and straight.
  - For sitting exercises, sit tall with your feet firmly on the floor.
- Perform each exercise slowly and smoothly.
- Do each exercise in a pain-free range of motion.
- Do not increase resistance too quickly.
- Begin with a warm-up session.
- End with the warm-down stretching exercises.

Safety Reminders
- Do not hold your breath while exercising.
- Stop immediately if you are short of breath.
- Stop immediately if you become fatigued.
- Exercises should not cause pain.

WARM-UP EXERCISES

The purpose of the warm-up is to increase blood flow to key muscle groups just before strength training. The warm-up takes four to five minutes. Any fairly vigorous activity can be substituted for this warm-up as long as it is done just before the strengthening exercises and it increases your heart rate slightly.

Gently and steadily perform the described movements for the designated time. When you are done, your heart rate should be slightly faster, and you should be breathing slightly harder. You should not feel fatigued. If you do, stop immediately.

Arm Swings

Stand with proper posture.

1
Swing one arm back and forth for 30 to 60 seconds.

2
Swing your other arm back and forth for 30 to 60 seconds.

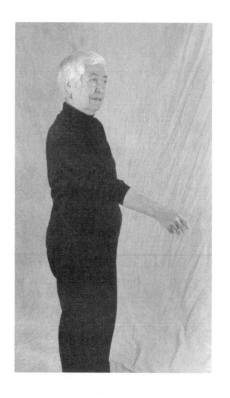

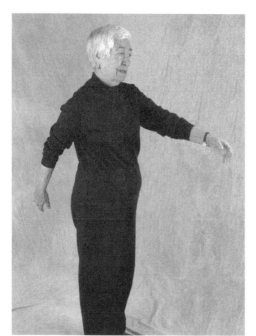

3
Swing both arms, alternating one forward and one backward, for 60 seconds.

Leg Swings

Stand with proper posture. Steady yourself with one hand on the back of a sturdy chair and keep your trunk still throughout the exercise.

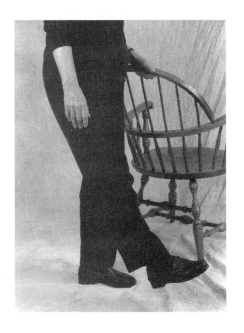 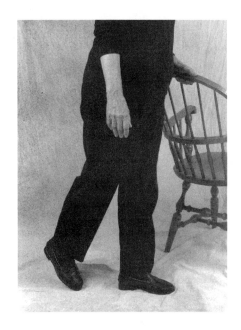

1
Swing one leg back and forth for 60 seconds.

2
Swing your other leg back and forth for 60 seconds.

This completes your warm-up. You are now ready to start the strength-training exercises.

STRENGTHENING EXERCISES

The General Strength Training program includes thirteen exercises for key muscle groups in your arms, legs, and trunk. If an exercise causes pain, limit your range of motion during that exercise. For example, if it hurts to straighten your leg, don't straighten it all the way. If you still have pain while limiting the motion, do not do the exercise.

Some exercises call for a length of resistance band. Others call for a loop of band. To make a loop, tie the ends of the band together. You may want to exercise without a band at first, adding it only when you feel ready.

For exercises without a Thera-Band exercise band:
- Begin with 10 repetitions.
- As the exercises get easier, progress to 12 and then to 15 repetitions.
- Next, progress to two sets of 10, then 12, then 15 repetitions.
- Finally, if able, progress to three sets of 10, then 12, then 15 repetitions.

For exercises with a Thera-Band exercise band:
- Begin with 10 repetitions.
- As the exercises get easier, progress to 12 and then to 15 repetitions.
- Next, move to a higher level band and do 10, then 12, then 15 repetitions.
- After you reach your ideal level of resistance, do two sets of 10, then 12, then 15.
- Finally, if able, progress to three sets of 10, then 12, then 15 repetitions.

Heel Lifts—Both Feet

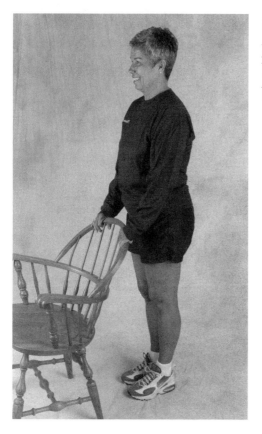

Stand with proper posture and place both hands on the back of a sturdy chair.

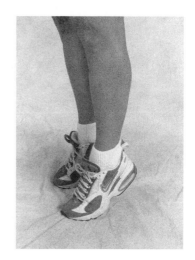

1
Raise both heels off the floor.

2
Feel the muscles working in your ankles and calves.

3
Slowly lower your heels to the ground. Repeat 10 times.

When this exercise becomes too easy, go on to the next exercise—heel lifts with one foot.

Heel Lifts–One Foot

Do this exercise only after heel lifts become too easy with
both feet.

With proper posture, stand on one foot and place
both hands on the back of a sturdy chair.

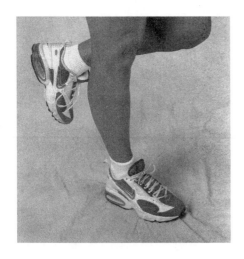 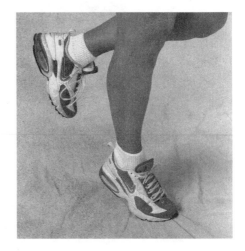

1
Raise your heel off the floor.

2
Feel the muscles working in your ankle and calf.

3
Slowly lower your heel to the ground. Repeat 10
times with each foot.

Leg Lifts
(use a loop of resistance band)

Sit with proper posture and loop the band around your ankles.

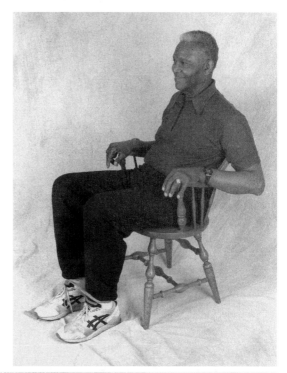

1
Leave one foot on the floor and slowly straighten your other leg against the band's resistance.

2
Feel the muscles working in the front of your thigh.

3
Slowly lower your foot back to the floor. Repeat 10 times with each leg.

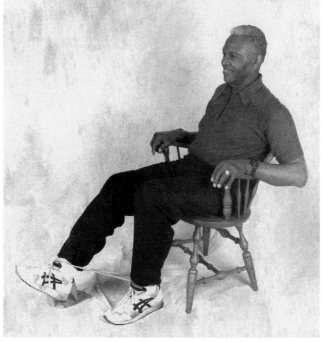

Thigh Lifts
(use a loop of resistance band)

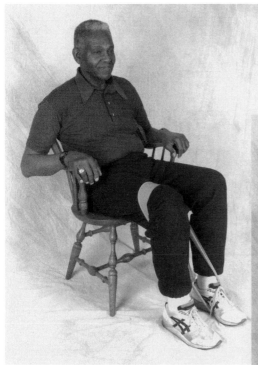

Sit with proper posture and place the loop under one foot and around the opposite knee.

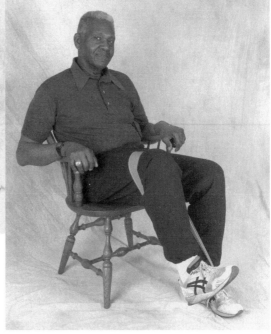

1
Lift your thigh off the chair against the band's resistance.

2
Feel the muscles working in your hip and thigh.

3
Slowly return to the starting position. Repeat 10 times with each leg.

Backward Leg Pulls
(use a loop of resistance band)

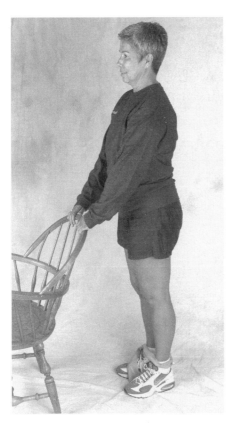

Stand with proper posture. Place both hands on the back of a sturdy chair. Loop the band around both ankles.

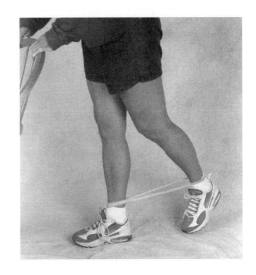

1
While keeping one foot firmly on the floor, tighten your buttocks and pull the band backward with your opposite foot.

2
Feel the muscles working in your hip and thigh.

3
Slowly return to the starting position. Repeat 10 times with each leg.

Side Leg Lifts
(use a loop of resistance band)

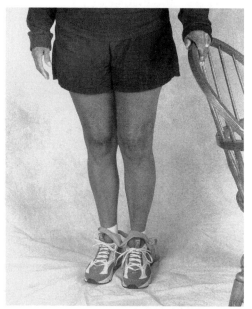

Stand sideways, feet together, with one hand on the back of a sturdy chair. Loop the band around both ankles. Keep the foot nearest the chair firmly on the floor, with the knee slightly bent. Maintain proper posture throughout the exercise.

1

Tighten your buttocks and slowly pull the band out to the side. (Keep your feet pointed straight ahead.)

2

Feel the muscles working along the side of your hip and thigh.

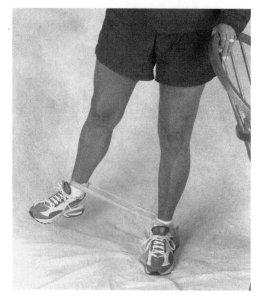

3

Slowly return your leg to the starting position. Repeat 10 times with each leg.

Side Leg Pulls
(use a loop of resistance band)

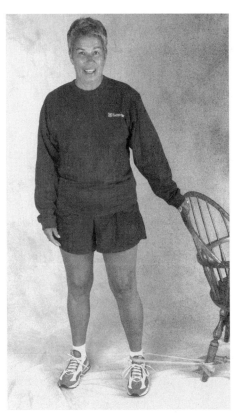

Stand sideways in a wide stance with one hand on the back of a sturdy chair. Loop the band around the chair leg and the ankle nearest the chair. Maintain proper posture throughout the exercise.

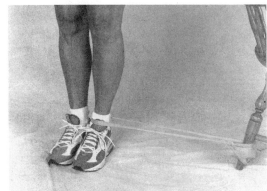

1
Pull the band away from the chair, bringing your feet together.

2
Feel the muscles working along your inner thigh.

3
Slowly return to the starting position. Repeat 10 times with each leg.

Forward Curls
(use a length of resistance band)

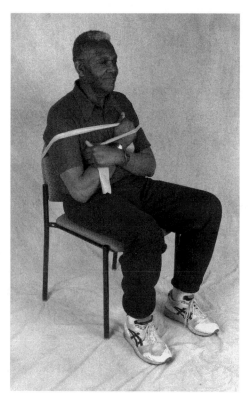

Sit with proper posture and loop the band around the back of the chair. Grasp each end of the band and cross your arms.

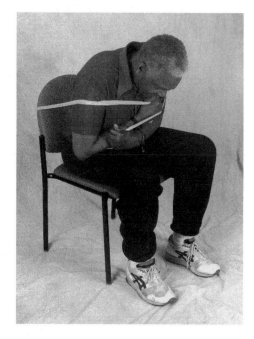

1
Curl your head and shoulders down toward your lap until your elbows touch your thighs.

2
Concentrate on contracting your abdominal muscles against the band's resistance.

3
Slowly return to the starting position. Repeat 10 times.

Arm Pumps
(use a length of resistance band)

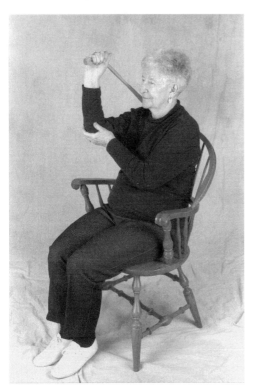

With proper posture, sit on one end of the band and bring the other over your shoulder, grasping it from behind. Bend your arm and raise your elbow to shoulder level. Use your other hand to support your elbow.

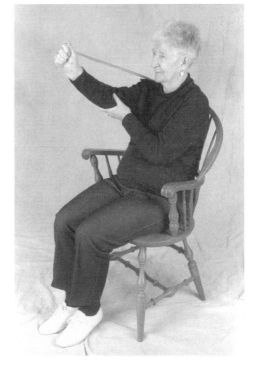

1
Keeping your elbow stationary, straighten your arm in front of you.

2
Feel the muscles working in your upper arm.

3
Slowly return to the starting position. Repeat 10 times with each arm.

Arm Curls
(use a length of resistance band)

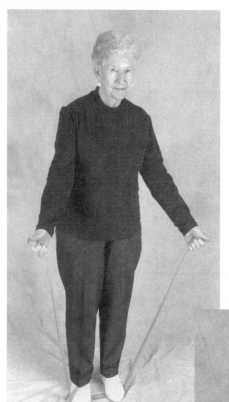

Stand on the band, grasping each end with your palms facing forward. Maintain proper posture.

1

Keeping your elbows stationary and close to your body, bend your arms and bring your hands toward your shoulders, palms up. (Keep your upper body still.)

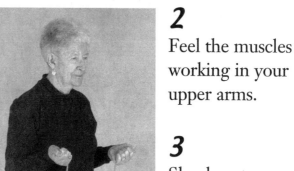

2

Feel the muscles working in your upper arms.

3

Slowly return to the starting position. Repeat 10 times.

Upper Back Builder
(use a length of resistance band)

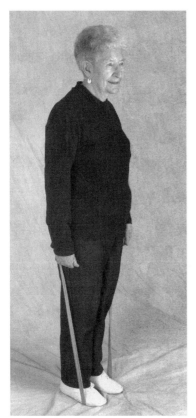

Stand on the band, grasping each end with your palms facing inward. Maintain proper posture.

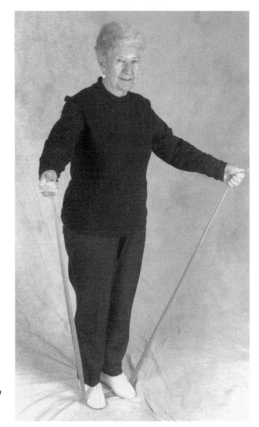

1
With elbows slightly bent, raise your arms along a 45-degree angle, staying below shoulder level.

2
Feel the muscles working in your shoulders and upper back.

3
Slowly return to the starting position. Repeat 10 times.

"Cross Country" Skiing
(use a length of resistance band)

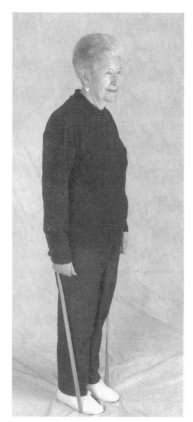

Stand on the band, grasping each end with your palms facing inward. Tighten your abdominal muscles and maintain proper posture.

1

Bring one arm forward and the other arm behind.

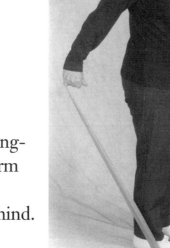

2

Now switch, bringing your other arm forward and the opposite arm behind.

3

Feel the muscles working in your shoulders. Repeat 10 times.

Shoulder Blade Squeeze
(use a length of resistance band)

Stand with proper posture. Grasp the band with both hands and raise your elbows to shoulder level, pointing them out to the sides.

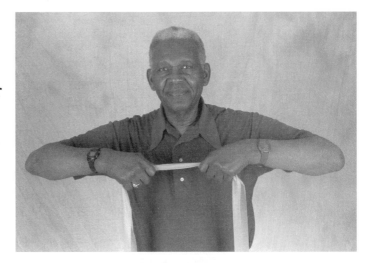

1

Pull your hands apart, squeezing your shoulder blades together.

2

Slowly return to the starting position. Repeat 10 times.

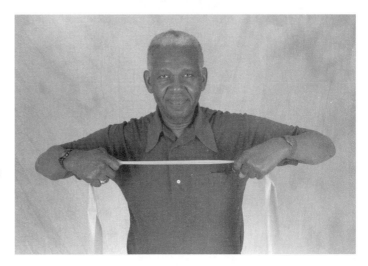

This completes your strengthening exercises. You are now ready to "warm down" with some stretching exercises.

WARM-DOWN STRETCHING EXERCISES

A gentle stretching session is the perfect way to "warm down." Stretching also makes your joints and muscles more flexible. In fact, stretching has been shown to decrease many aches and pains associated with advancing age.

Ease into each stretch until you feel a gentle pull or tug along the muscle. Do not bounce. You should not feel pain. If you do, review the technique for the stretch and try again. If you still have pain, leave that particular stretch out of your routine.

Perform each stretch twice, holding for twenty seconds. Do all stretches while standing tall and straight, your ears aligned with your shoulders.

Neck Stretch

Stand with proper posture.

1

Tilt your head to the side, moving your ear toward your shoulder.

2

Feel the stretch along the side of your neck.

3

Hold for 20 seconds.

4

Return your head to an upright position. Do the stretch 2 times on each side.

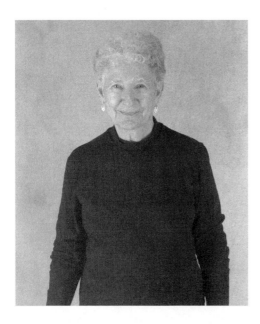 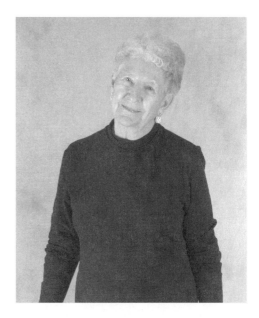

Shoulder Stretch—over the Head

Stand with proper posture. Place one hand at the back of your neck, pointing your elbow in the air.

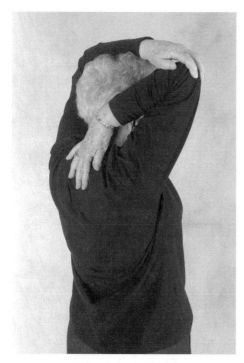

1

Using your other hand, gently pull your elbow toward the middle of your back.

2

Feel the stretch along your shoulder.

3

Hold for 20 seconds.

4

Release the stretch briefly. Do the stretch 2 times with each arm.

Shoulder Stretch—across the Body

Stand with proper posture. Bring one arm across your body, resting your hand on your shoulder.

1
Using your other hand, gently pull your elbow farther across your body.

2
Feel the stretch along the back of your shoulder.

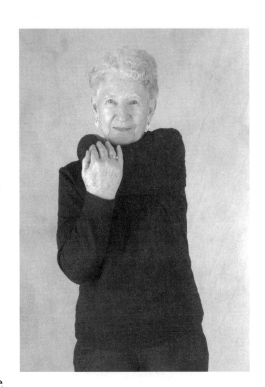

3
Hold for 20 seconds.

4
Release the stretch briefly. Do the stretch 2 times with each arm.

Chest Stretch

Stand with proper posture and clasp your hands behind your back.

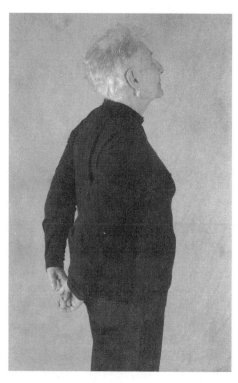

1

Gently pull your shoulder blades down and together, lifting up through your chest.

2

Feel this stretch along the front of your shoulders and chest.

3

Hold for 20 seconds.

4

Release the stretch briefly. Repeat.

Calf Stretch

Stand with your hands on the back of a sturdy chair. Place one foot behind your body, keeping the leg straight. Maintain proper posture throughout the exercise.

1

With your toes pointing straight ahead and your heels flat on the floor, gently lunge forward.

2

Feel the stretch in your calf.

3

Hold for 20 seconds.

4

Release the stretch briefly. Do the stretch 2 times with each leg.

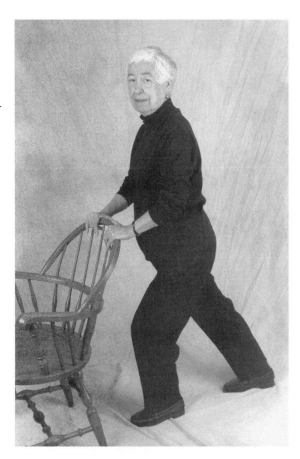

Hamstring Stretch

Stand with proper posture and place one hand on the back of a sturdy chair. Set one foot on the seat of a chair or stool.

1

Keeping your back straight, lean forward at your waist, being careful not to stretch too far and lose proper form.

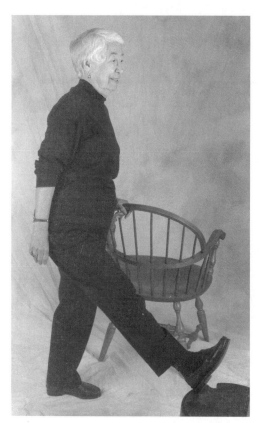

2

Feel the gentle stretch along the back of your thigh.

3

Hold for 20 seconds.

4

Release the stretch briefly. Do the stretch 2 times with each leg.

Thigh Stretch

Stand with proper posture and place one hand on the back of a sturdy chair.

1

Grasp one foot and bring the heel to your buttocks; do not bend at the waist.

2

Feel the stretch along the front of your thigh.

3

Hold for 20 seconds.

4

Release the stretch briefly. Do the stretch 2 times with each leg.

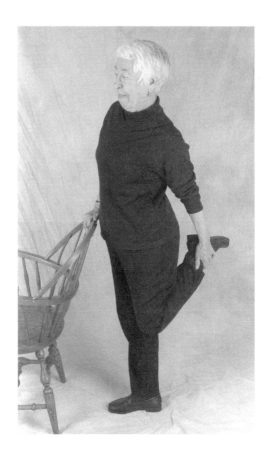

Inner Thigh Stretch

Stand with proper posture and place one hand on the back of a sturdy chair. Set your feet in a wide stance.

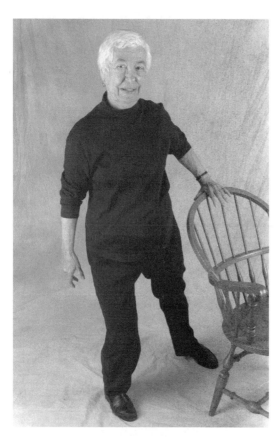

1
Bend one knee and lunge to the side.

2
Feel the stretch in the inner thigh of your opposite leg.

3
Hold for 20 seconds.

4
Release the stretch briefly. Do the stretch 2 times with each leg.

CONCLUSION

The General Strength Training program is designed to strengthen all the major muscle groups in your body. It will help you counter your body's tendency to grow weaker as you age. The stronger your muscles, the more likely you are to maintain an independent lifestyle and enjoy good health now and in the years ahead.

Kecia E. Sell is the manager of clinical operations for the Clinical/Quality Systems Division of Fairview Rehabilitation Services, as well as a physical therapist in the hospitals and outpatient clinics within the Fairview system. Ms. Sell received her BA degree from Gustavus Adolphus College in St. Peter, Minnesota, and her MS degree in physical therapy from the Krannert Graduate School of Physical Therapy at the University of Indianapolis. Kecia and her husband, Jim, have one son, Jordan.

Lorie A. Schleck is a physical therapist at Fairview Rehabilitation Services. She received her BS degree in physical therapy from the University of Minnesota and her MA degree in counseling psychology from St. Mary's University of Minnesota. Lorie and her husband, Jim, have a son, Ben, and a daughter, Kara.

4

Osteoporosis Prevention

Elizabeth Smith, PT, ATC/R
Lorie A. Schleck, MA, PT

This program takes about 30 minutes.
Do it 2 to 3 times each week.
A 48-hour break is recommended between each session.

EQUIPMENT NEEDED:
   Stable, heavy chair that will not tip over
   Chair of stool
   Length of resistance band (3 to 4 feet)
   Loop of resistance band
   Rolled-up towel
   Door

Osteoporosis is a disease that makes our bones fragile and susceptible to fractures. It is sometimes called a "silent disease" because significant bone loss can occur without symptoms. Most people do not know they have osteoporosis until a sudden bump, strain, or fall causes a weak bone to break. Such fractures are a source of fear, pain, and disability.

RISK FACTORS

Some of us are at greater risk for developing osteoporosis than others. The National Osteoporosis Foundation has identified several "risk factors" that might increase our chances of developing this disease.

Risk Factors for Osteoporosis

Gender (female)
Advancing age
Caffeine use
Alcohol use
Calcium-deficient diet
Smoking
Family history of
   osteoporosis
Race (Asian or
   Caucasian)
Thin or small frame
Menopause
   (including surgically
   induced menopause)
Inactive lifestyle

One of the most important risk factors is gender. While osteoporosis strikes one out of eight men over age 50, women are four times more likely than men to develop the disease. In fact, over half of 50-year-old women are expected to have a fracture related to osteoporosis in their lifetime.

One reason for this gender difference is that women build less bone density in their youth. Therefore, as adults, women's bones aren't as strong as men's. Menopause is another factor: When menopause occurs, women experience a significant decrease in estrogen production, which causes accelerated bone loss.

But gender isn't the only risk factor. Age, race, diet, health habits, certain medications, and some diseases may also increase a person's chances of developing osteoporosis. The best way to determine your risk is to talk to your doctor about your health history and other risk factors.

Prevention

There is no cure for osteoporosis. But for most people, osteoporosis can be prevented. True, we cannot change our gender or reverse the aging process. But we can quit smoking, exercise more, drink less caffeine and alcohol, and add more calcium to our diet. While these steps may not completely eliminate the risk of osteoporosis, they can help ensure stronger, healthier bones.

According to the National Osteoporosis Foundation, a complete osteoporosis prevention program has four parts:

1. A balanced diet with adequate amounts of calcium and vitamin D.

2. A healthy lifestyle that includes little or no alcohol and no smoking.

3. Medications and bone density testing, when appropriate.

4. Weight-bearing exercise, including strength training.

The strengthening exercises in this chapter may be used as part of a complete osteoporosis prevention program. Because strength training has been shown to slow or reverse bone loss, it is considered a critical lifestyle choice for anyone who hopes to prevent osteoporosis.

A recent study compared two groups of postmenopausal women averaging 54 years of age. One group participated in regular strength-training exercises, the other did not. After nine months, the women in the strength-training program experienced an average increase in bone density of 1.6 percent. The women who did not strength train experienced a bone *loss* of 3.6 percent. This study focused on the spine—an area particularly susceptible to osteoporotic fracture—but strength training also increases bone density in two other important areas: the hips and the wrists.

Strength-training exercises must be site specific: To strengthen your spine, you must exercise your back. Therefore, the exercises in this chapter focus specifically on areas where osteoporosis creates the greatest risk for fracture.

THE PROGRAM

This strengthening program consists of a warm-up session, strengthening exercises, and warm-down stretching exercises. The exercises are designed to build bone density by placing a certain amount of stress on your bones. You will also see an improvement in your posture and flexibility.

You may want to meet with a physical therapist or other healthcare professional before beginning this program. A trained professional can help make sure you are exercising properly.

Exercise Guidelines
- Wear comfortable, nonbinding clothing.
- Maintain proper body alignment:
  - For standing exercises, stand tall and straight.
  - For sitting exercises, sit tall with your feet firmly on the floor.
- Perform each exercise slowly and smoothly.
- Do each exercise in a pain-free range of motion.
- Do not increase resistance too quickly.
- Begin with a warm-up session.
- End with the warm-down stretching exercises.

Safety Reminders
- Do not hold your breath while exercising.
- Stop immediately if you are short of breath.
- Stop immediately if you become fatigued.
- Exercises should not cause pain.

WARM-UP EXERCISES

The purpose of the warm-up is to increase blood flow to key muscle groups just before strength training. The warm-up takes four to five minutes. Any fairly vigorous activity can be substituted for this warm-up as long as it is done just before the strengthening exercises and it increases your heart rate slightly.

Gently and steadily perform the described movements for the designated time. When you are done, your heart rate should be slightly faster, and you should be breathing slightly harder. You should not feel fatigued. If you do, stop immediately.

Arm Swings

Stand with proper posture.

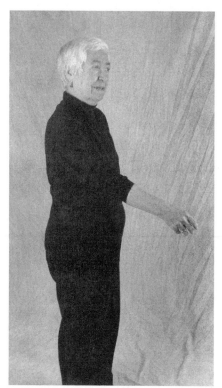

1

Swing one arm back and forth for 30 to 60 seconds.

2

Swing your other arm back and forth for 30 to 60 seconds.

3

Swing both arms, alternating one forward and one backward, for 60 seconds.

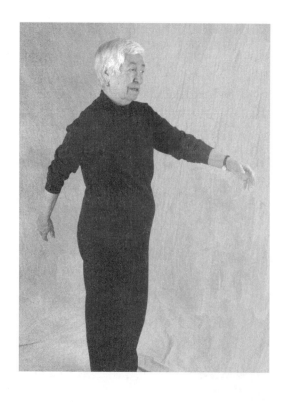

Leg Swings

Stand with proper posture. Steady yourself with one hand on the back of a sturdy chair and keep your trunk still throughout the exercise.

1

Swing one leg back and forth for 60 seconds.

2

Swing your other leg back and forth for 60 seconds.

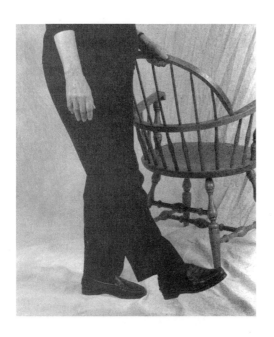 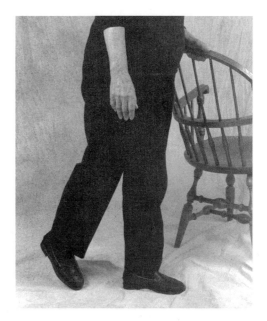

This completes your warm-up. You are now ready to start the strength-training exercises.

STRENGTHENING EXERCISES

The Osteoporosis Prevention program includes fifteen exercises for key muscle groups, including those affecting the spine, hips, and wrists. If an exercise causes pain, limit your range of motion during that exercise. For example, if it hurts to straighten your leg, don't straighten it all the way. If you still have pain while limiting the motion, do not do the exercise.

Some exercises call for a length of resistance band. Others call for a loop of band. To make a loop, tie the ends of the band together. You may want to exercise without a band at first, adding it only when you feel ready.

For exercises without a Thera-Band resistance band:
- Begin with 10 repetitions.
- As the exercises get easier, progress to 12 and then to 15 repetitions.
- Next, progress to two sets of 10, then 12, then 15 repetitions.
- Finally, if able, progress to three sets of 10, then 12, then 15 repetitions.

For exercises with a Thera-Band resistance band:
- Begin with 10 repetitions.
- As the exercises get easier, progress to 12 and then to 15 repetitions.
- Next, move to a higher level band and do 10, then 12, then 15 repetitions.
- After you reach your ideal level of resistance, do two sets of 10, then 12, then 15.
- Finally, if able, progress to three sets of 10, then 12, then 15 repetitions.

Two-Leg Squat
(use a length of resistance band)

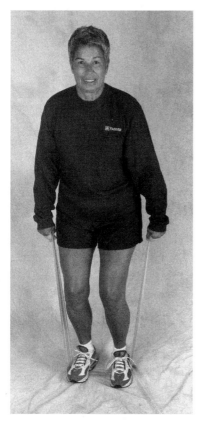

Stand on the band with your knees bent. Grasp each end and pull the band taut. Maintain an upright posture throughout the exercise.

1
Straighten your knees slowly against the band's resistance.

2
Pause briefly at the top, keeping your knees slightly bent.

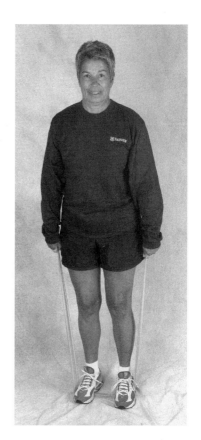

3
Feel the muscles working along the front of your thighs.

4
Slowly return to the starting position. Repeat 10 times.

When the two-leg squat becomes too easy, no matter how much resistance you add, progress to the next exercise—the one-leg squat.

One-Leg Squat
(use a length of resistance band)

Do this exercise only after the two-leg squat becomes too easy.

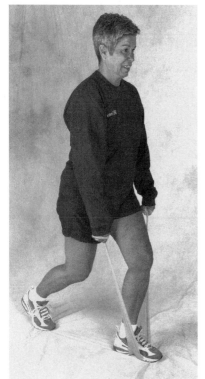

Put your right foot forward and bend your knees. Place the band under your right foot, grasp each end, and pull the band taut. Be sure to maintain an upright posture throughout the exercise.

1

Straighten your knee slowly against the band's resistance.

2

Pause briefly at the top, keeping your knee slightly bent.

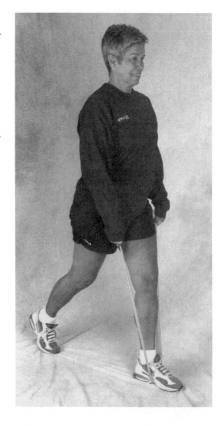

3

Feel the muscle working along the front of your thigh.

4

Slowly return to the starting position. Repeat 10 times with each leg.

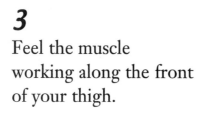

Heel Lifts—Both Feet

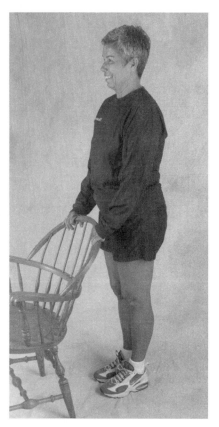

Stand with proper posture and place both hands on the back of a sturdy chair.

1
Raise both heels off the floor.

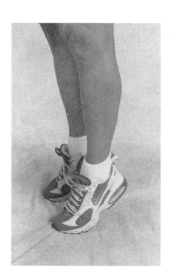

2
Feel the muscles working in your ankles and calves.

3
Slowly lower your heels to the ground. Repeat 10 times.

When this exercise becomes too easy, go on to the next exercise—heel lifts with one foot.

Heel Lifts—One Foot

Do this exercise only after heel lifts become too easy with both feet.

With proper posture, stand on one foot and place both hands on the back of a sturdy chair.

1
Raise your heel off the floor.

2
Feel the muscles working in your ankle and calf.

3
Slowly lower your heel to the ground. Repeat 10 times with each foot.

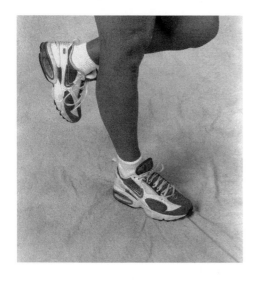 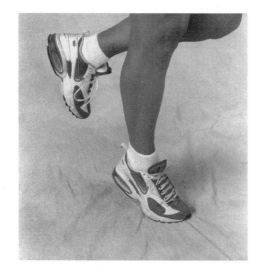

Backward Leg Pulls
(use a loop of resistance band)

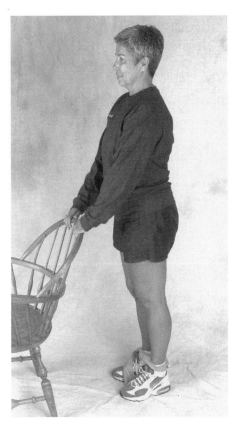

Stand with proper posture. Place both hands on the back of a sturdy chair. Loop the band around both ankles.

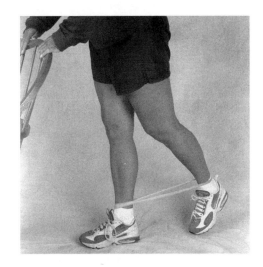

1

While keeping one foot firmly on the floor, tighten your buttocks and pull the band backward with your opposite foot.

2

Feel the muscles working in your hip and thigh.

3

Slowly return to the starting position. Repeat 10 times with each leg.

Side Leg Lifts
(use a loop of resistance band)

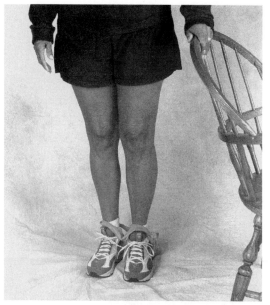

Stand sideways, feet together, with one hand on the back of a sturdy chair. Loop the band around both ankles. Keep the foot nearest the chair firmly on the floor, with the knee slightly bent. Maintain proper posture throughout the exercise.

1
Tighten your buttocks and slowly pull the band out to the side. (Keep your feet pointed straight ahead.)

2
Feel the muscles working along the side of your hip and thigh.

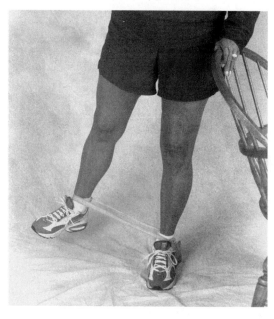

3
Slowly return your leg to the starting position. Repeat 10 times with each leg.

Side Leg Pulls
(use a loop of resistance band)

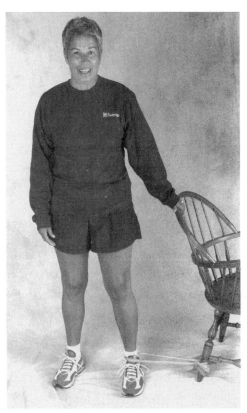

Stand sideways in a wide stance with one hand on the back of a sturdy chair. Loop the band around one chair leg and the ankle nearest the chair. Maintain an upright posture throughout the exercise.

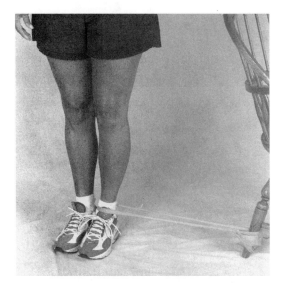

1
Pull the band away from the chair, bringing your feet together.

2
Feel the muscles working along your inner thigh.

3
Slowly return to the starting position. Repeat 10 times with each leg.

Pull-Downs
(use a length of resistance band)

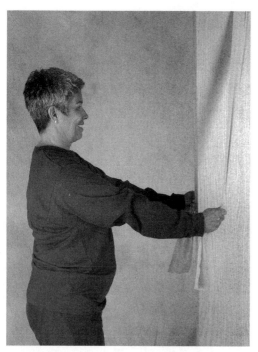

Drape the band over the top of an open door (4 to 6 inches from the door's edge, so it doesn't slip). Grasp each end, keeping your arms straight.

1
Squeezing your shoulder blades together, pull the band down to your thighs. (Keep your elbows close to your body.)

2
Feel the muscles working in your upper back and shoulders.

3
Slowly return to the starting position. Repeat 10 times.

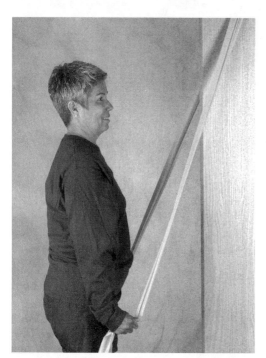

Arm Pumps
(use a length of resistance band)

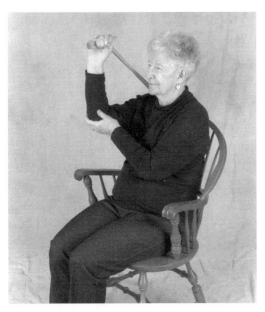

With proper posture, sit on one end of the band and bring the other end over your shoulder, grasping it from behind. Bend your arm and raise your elbow to shoulder level. Support your elbow with your other hand.

1
Keeping your elbow stationary, straighten your arm in front of you.

2
Feel the muscles working in your upper arm.

3
Slowly return to the starting position. Repeat 10 times with each arm.

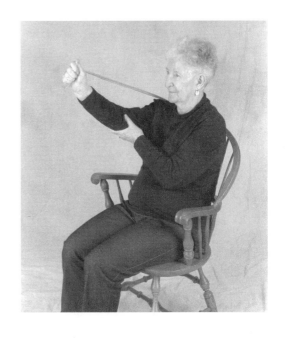

Arm Curls
(use a length of resistance band)

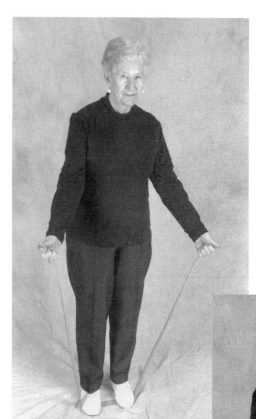

Stand on the band, grasping each end with your palms facing forward. Maintain proper posture.

1

Keeping your elbows stationary and close to your body, bend your arms and bring your hands toward your shoulders, palms up. (Keep your upper body still.)

2

Feel the muscles working in your upper arms.

3

Slowly return to the starting position. Repeat 10 times.

Wrist Curls—Palm Up
(use a length of resistance band)

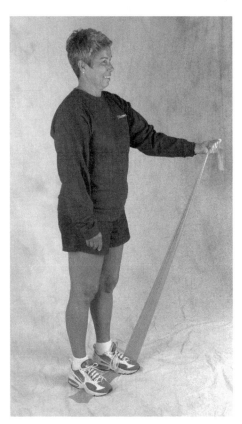

Stand on one end of the band and grasp the other end in one hand, palm up. Hold your forearm steady. Keep your elbow slightly bent and at your side throughout the exercise. Maintain proper posture.

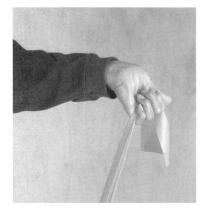

1
Slowly bend your wrist backward and down.

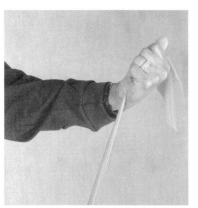

2
Slowly curl it up. Repeat 10 times with each wrist.

Wrist Curls—Palm Down
(use a length of resistance band)

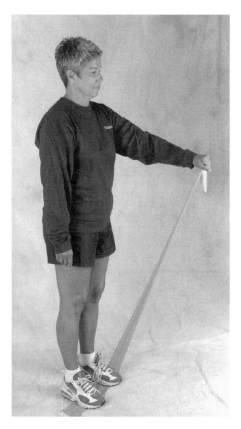

Stand on one end of the band and grasp the other end in one hand, palm down. Hold your forearm steady. Keep your elbow slightly bent and at your side throughout the exercise. Maintain proper posture.

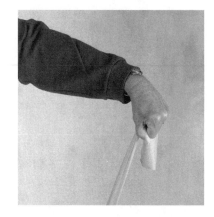

1
Slowly curl your wrist forward and down.

2
Slowly bend it up and back. Repeat 10 times with each wrist.

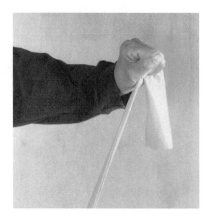

Trunk Lifts
(use a rolled-up towel)

Lie face down on the floor with your arms at your sides and your forehead resting on the towel.

1
Slowly raise your head and shoulders off the floor.

2
Pause at the top of the movement and feel the muscles working along your spine.

3
Slowly return to the floor. Repeat 10 times.

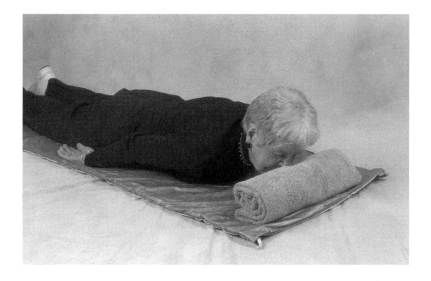

When this exercise becomes too easy, go on to the next exercise—trunk lifts using a Thera-Band resistance band.

Trunk Lifts—with a Band
(use a rolled-up towel)

Do this exercise only after trunk lifts become too easy without a band.

Lie face down on the floor with your forehead resting on the towel. Place the band across your upper back, holding an end in each hand. The band should be taut.

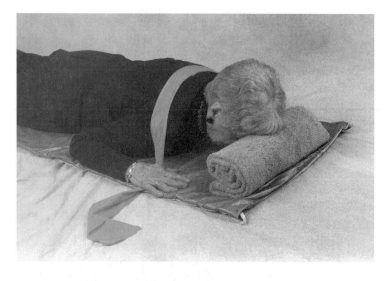

1
Lift your head and shoulders against the band's resistance.

2
Pause at the top of the movement and feel the muscles working along your spine.

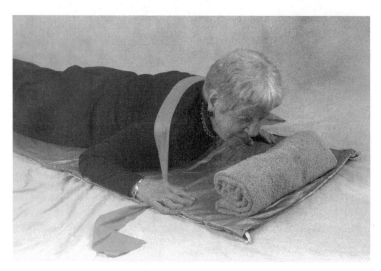

3
Slowly return to the floor. Repeat 10 times.

Side Bends
(use a length of resistance band)

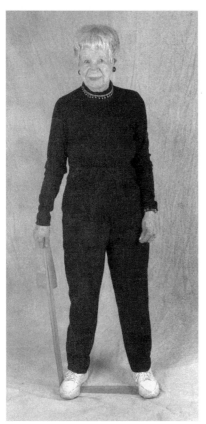

Stand on the band. Grasp one end of the band, maintaining proper posture.

1

Bend your trunk in the opposite direction, against the band's resistance. (Do not allow your trunk to rotate.)

2

Feel the muscles working along the side of your trunk.

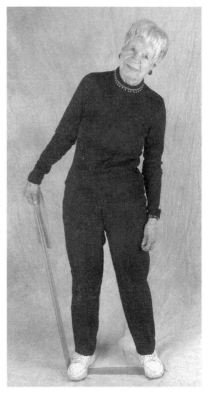

3

Return to the starting position. Repeat 10 times on each side.

This completes your strengthening exercises. You are now ready to "warm down" with some stretching exercises.

WARM-DOWN STRETCHING EXERCISES

A gentle stretching session is the perfect way to "warm down." Stretching also makes your joints and muscles more flexible. In fact, stretching has been shown to decrease many aches and pains associated with advancing age.

Ease into each stretch until you feel a gentle pull or tug along the muscle. Do not bounce. You should not feel pain. If you do, review the technique for the stretch and try again. If you still have pain, leave that particular stretch out of your routine.

Perform each stretch twice, holding for twenty seconds. Do all stretches while standing tall and straight, your ears aligned with your shoulders.

Neck Stretch

Stand with proper posture.

1

Tilt your head to the side, moving your ear toward your shoulder.

2

Feel the stretch along the side of your neck.

3

Hold for 20 seconds.

4

Return your head to an upright position. Do the stretch 2 times on each side.

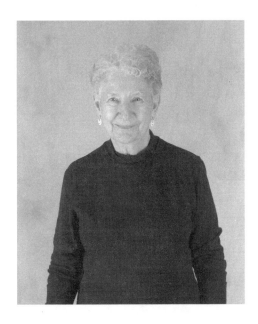
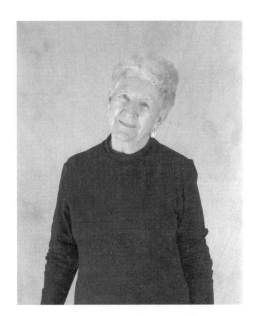

Shoulder Stretch—over the Head

Stand with proper posture. Place one hand at the
back of your neck, pointing your elbow in the air.

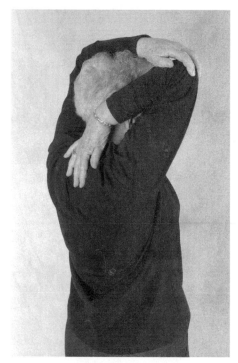

1

Using your other hand, gently pull
your elbow toward the middle of
your back.

2

Feel the stretch along your shoulder.

3

Hold for 20 seconds.

4

Release the stretch briefly. Do the
stretch 2 times with each arm.

Shoulder Stretch–across the Body

Stand with proper posture. Bring one arm across your body, resting your hand on your shoulder.

1

Using your other hand, gently pull your elbow farther across your body.

2

Feel the stretch along the back of your shoulder.

3

Hold for 20 seconds.

4

Release the stretch briefly. Do the stretch 2 times with each arm.

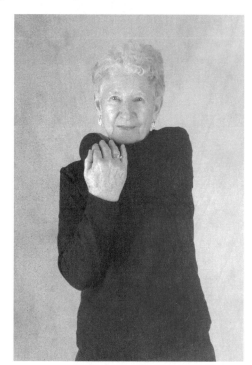

Chest Stretch

Stand with proper posture and clasp your hands behind your back.

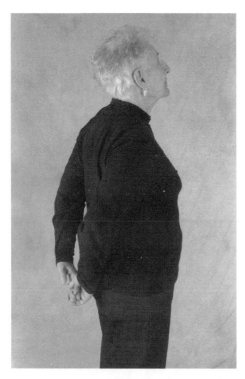

1

Gently pull your shoulder blades down and together, lifting up through your chest.

2

Feel this stretch along the front of your shoulders and chest.

3

Hold for 20 seconds.

4

Release the stretch briefly. Repeat.

Calf Stretch

Stand with your hands on the back of a sturdy chair. Place one foot behind your body, keeping the leg straight. Maintain proper posture throughout the exercise.

1

With your toes pointing straight ahead and your heels flat on the floor, gently lunge forward.

2

Feel the stretch in your calf.

3

Hold for 20 seconds.

4

Release the stretch briefly. Do the stretch 2 times with each leg.

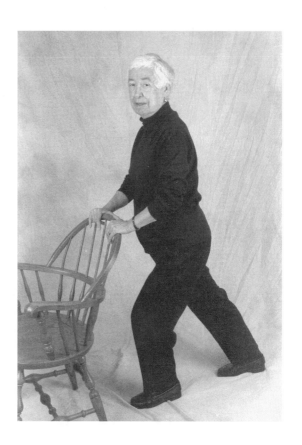

Hamstring Stretch

Stand with proper posture and place one hand on the back of a sturdy chair. Set one foot on the seat of a chair or stool.

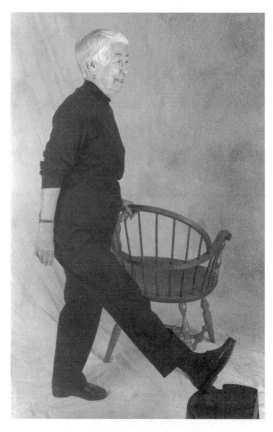

1
Keeping your back straight, lean forward at your waist, being careful not to stretch too far and lose proper form.

2
Feel the gentle stretch along the back of your thigh.

3
Hold for 20 seconds.

4
Release the stretch briefly. Do the stretch 2 times with each leg.

Thigh Stretch

Stand with proper posture and place one hand on the back of a sturdy chair.

1

Grasp one foot and bring the heel to your buttocks. Do not bend at the waist.

2

Feel the stretch along the front of your thigh.

3

Hold for 20 seconds.

4

Release the stretch briefly. Do the stretch 2 times with each leg.

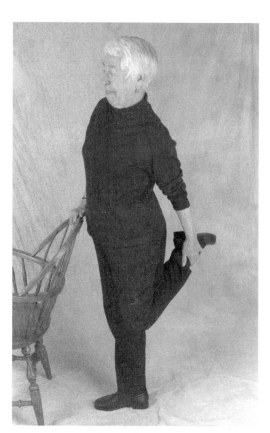

Inner Thigh Stretch

Stand with proper posture and place one hand on the back of a sturdy chair. Set your feet in a wide stance.

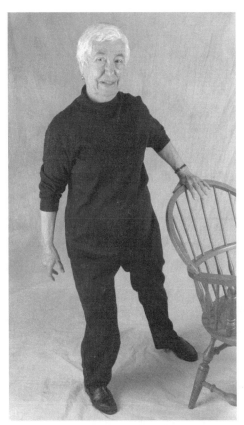

1

Bend one knee and lunge to the side.

2

Feel the stretch in the inner thigh of your opposite leg.

3

Hold for 20 seconds.

4

Release the stretch briefly. Repeat 2 times with each leg.

CONCLUSION

Osteoporosis can be debilitating. It can also be prevented. Strength training is just one part of a complete osteoporosis prevention program, but it is a very important part. The strength-training program outlined in this chapter is designed to specifically strengthen those parts of your body most susceptible to fracture when osteoporosis is present. Regular strength training can be your route to stronger bones and muscles.

Elizabeth Smith received degrees in athletic training and physical therapy from the University of Wisconsin, Madison. She supervises an outpatient clinic for Fairview Rehabilitation Services and provides care to a variety of patients. She specializes in evaluating and designing exercise programs for patients with osteoporosis and those predisposed to this condition. Elizabeth and her husband, Kevin, live in St. Paul.

Lorie A. Schleck is a physical therapist at Fairview Rehabilitation Services. She received her BS degree in physical therapy from the University of Minnesota and her MA degree in counseling psychology from St. Mary's University of Minnesota. Lorie and her husband, Jim, have a son, Ben, and a daughter, Kara.

Strength Training with Osteoporosis

Elizabeth Smith, PT, ATC/R
Lorie A. Schleck, MA, PT

All three phases of this program take only 30 minutes.
Do Phases I and II daily. Do Phase III every other day.

EQUIPMENT NEEDED:
  Stable, heavy chair that will not tip over
  Railing, kitchen sink, or heavy piece of furniture
  Length of resistance band (3 to 4 feet)
  Loop of resistance band
  Small cuff weights (optional)

If you have been diagnosed with osteoporosis, you are at risk for having a fracture. Those of us with osteoporosis must approach strength training differently. To prevent injury, we must be aware of every movement we make, and we must understand which movements are safe and which are unsafe.

It is possible to exercise safely. In fact, we need to begin exercising as soon as we are able. Inactivity and lack of exercise accelerate bone loss. A strength-training program, properly employed, can help reduce the risks of falling and of further bone loss through increased muscle strength, flexibility, and coordination.

PRECAUTIONS

If you have osteoporosis, you must take several safety precautions when strength training:

• **Talk with your doctor.** Because your physician has specific knowledge of your medical history, he or she can best judge the safety and benefits of a strength-training program.

• **Avoid bending forward from your waist with a rounded back.** This movement increases your chance of spinal fracture. Toe touches and sit-ups, for example, cause your spine to bend forward or become rounded—movements like these should be avoided.

• **Avoid any activity or exercise that jars your spine or creates a risk of falling.**

• **Do not perform any exercise that requires you to move your leg sideways away from your body or across your body.** These movements cause stress in the hip and may make a weakened hip susceptible to fracture.

THE PROGRAM

The exercises in this chapter are divided into three phases. Unless you're experiencing pain from a recent fracture, you can probably do all three phases from the start. If an exercise causes pain, limit your range of motion during that exercise. For example, if it hurts to straighten your leg, don't straighten it all the way. If you still have pain while limiting the motion, do not do the exercise.

Phase I includes some simple but extremely important exercises for your upper back and for improved spinal alignment. If you have had a spinal fracture and are still having significant pain, do only Phase I exercises until you feel well enough to progress to Phase II.

Phase II exercises are for the abdominal and back muscles. Begin Phase II when you are able. Do both Phase I and Phase II exercises daily.

Phase III exercises, for the arms and legs, complete the Strength Training with Osteoporosis program. Do Phase III exercises every other day.

Phase I is an adequate warm-up for the strength-training exercises in Phases II and III. After you complete the strengthening exercises, "warm down" through the gentle stretches outlined at the end of this chapter.

You may want to meet with a physical therapist or other healthcare professional before beginning this program. A trained professional can help make sure you are exercising properly.

Exercise Guidelines
- Wear comfortable, nonbinding clothing.
- Maintain proper body alignment:
  - For standing exercises, stand tall and straight.
  - For sitting exercises, sit tall with your feet firmly on the floor.
- Perform each exercise slowly and smoothly.
- Do each exercise in a pain-free range of motion.
- Do not increase resistance too quickly.
- End with the warm-down stretching exercises.

Safety Reminders
- Talk to your doctor before beginning this program.
- Do not hold your breath while exercising.
- Stop immediately if you are short of breath.
- Stop immediately if you become fatigued.
- Do not bend forward at your waist with a rounded spine.
- Avoid exercises that jar your spine.
- Do not move your leg sideways away from or across your body.
- Avoid slippery floors.
- Wear proper shoes to prevent falling.
- Exercises should not cause pain.

PHASE 1—WARM-UP EXERCISES

These exercises stretch your upper back and promote good spine alignment. Do them daily.

Upper Arm Press

Sit with proper posture, shoulders relaxed. Bend your elbows and keep them close to your body.

1

Push your upper arms into the back of the chair.

2

Hold for 5 seconds.

3

Relax. Repeat 10 times.

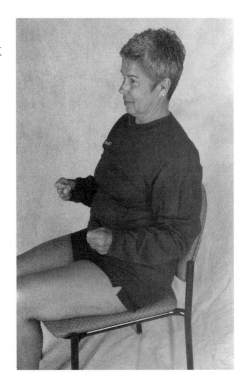

"Butterfly" Stretch

Sit with proper posture and place your hands behind your neck.

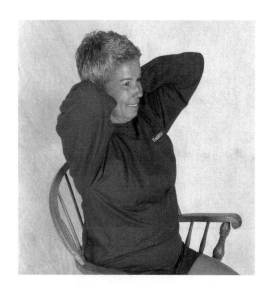 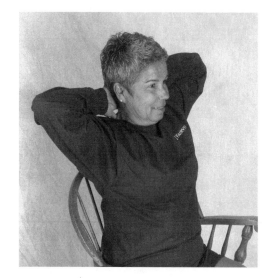

1

Slowly and gently bring your elbows backward, being careful not to pull on your neck.

2

When your elbows are as far back as they will go, pause briefly.

3

Feel the stretch in your shoulders and chest.

4

Relax and return to the starting position. Repeat 10 times.

Chest Stretch

Stand with proper posture and clasp your hands behind your back.

1

Gently pull your shoulder blades down and together, lifting up through your chest.

2

Feel this stretch along the front of your shoulders and chest.

3

Hold for 20 seconds.

4

Release the stretch briefly. Repeat.

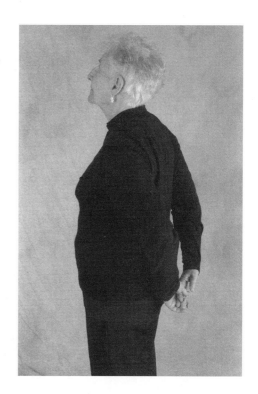

PHASE II EXERCISES

These exercises help strengthen your back and stomach muscles. Do the exercises daily.

Abdominal Press

Lie flat on the floor, face up, with your knees bent. Place your hands on your stomach.

1

Tighten your stomach muscles while flattening your back against the floor.

2

Feel with your hands as your stomach muscles tighten.

3

Hold for 5 seconds.

4

Release. Repeat 10 times.

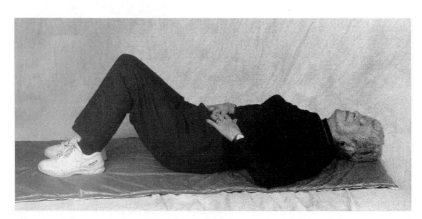

As you are able, work up to two or three sets of repetitions.

Arm Lifts

Get on your hands and knees. Keep your spine straight throughout this exercise—do not allow your back to sag or become rounded.

1
Tighten your abdominal muscles.

2
Lift one arm in front of you, pointing your thumb toward the ceiling.

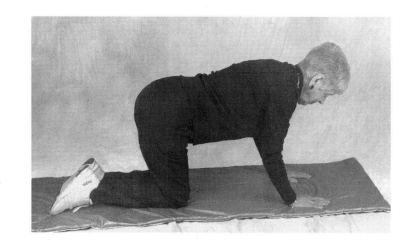

3
Lower your arm to the floor. Lift the other arm in front of you, pointing your thumb toward the ceiling. Repeat 10 times.

As this exercise gets easier, do two or three sets, or add cuff weights for resistance.

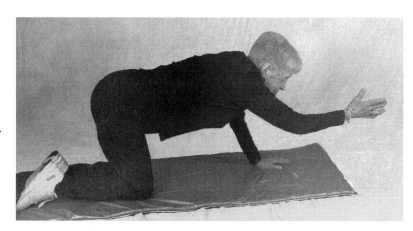

Leg Lifts

Get on your hands and knees. Keep the spine straight—do not allow your lower back to sag during the exercise.

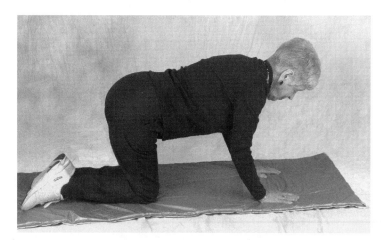

1
Tighten your abdominal muscles and keep your trunk still.

2
Lift one leg behind you.

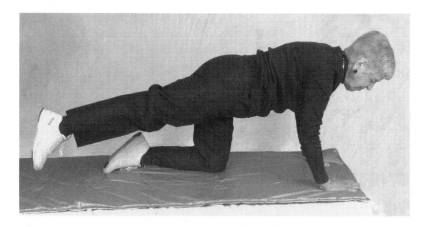

3
Lower your leg to the floor, then lift the other leg behind you. Repeat 10 times.

As this exercise gets easier, do two or three sets, or add cuff weights for resistance.

When arm lifts and leg lifts become too easy, even with resistance, go on to the next exercise—arm and leg lifts.

Arm and Leg Lifts

Do this exercise only after the arm lifts and leg lifts become too easy.

Get on your hands and knees. Keep your spine straight—do not allow your lower back to sag during this exercise.

1
Tighten your abdominal muscles.

2
Simultaneously lift one arm and the opposite leg.

3
Return to the starting position.

4
Simultaneously lift the other arm and opposite leg. Repeat 10 times.

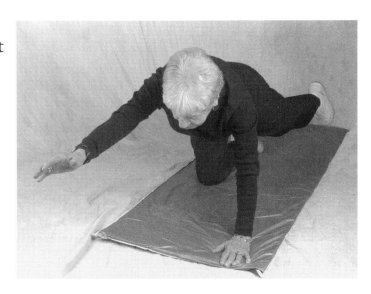

PHASE III EXERCISES

Phase III includes eight exercises to strengthen your arms and legs. Do them every other day.

If you're recovering from a fracture, some exercises may be too painful. That's okay. Just concentrate on the exercises you're able to do and add the others when you feel ready. Remember, it's important to resume (or begin) a complete strength-training program as soon as possible.

Some exercises call for a length of resistance band. Others call for a loop of band. To make a loop, tie the ends of the band together. You may want to exercise without a band at first, adding it only when you feel ready.

For exercises without a Thera-Band resistance band:
- Begin with 10 repetitions.
- As the exercises get easier, progress to 12 and then to 15 repetitions.
- Next, progress to two sets of 10, then 12, then 15 repetitions.
- Finally, if able, progress to three sets of 10, then 12, then 15 repetitions.

For exercises with a Thera-Band resistance band:
- Begin with 10 repetitions.
- As the exercises get easier, progress to 12 and then to 15 repetitions.
- Next, move to a higher level band and do 10, then 12, then 15 repetitions.
- After you reach your ideal level of resistance, do two sets of 10, then 12, then 15.
- Finally, if able, progress to three sets of 10, then 12, then 15 repetitions.

Half-Squat

Stand with proper posture and set your feet shoulder-width apart. Hold on to something firm at about waist height, like a railing, a heavy piece of furniture, the kitchen sink, or another person.

1
Bend your knees.

2
Slowly lower your body as if you were sitting down into a chair.

3
When you're partway down (about a quarter of the way), pause briefly.

4
Slowly return to the starting position, pushing up through your heels as you do so.

5
Throughout the movement, concentrate on using the muscles along the front of your thighs and your buttocks. Repeat 10 times.

Backward Leg Pulls
(use a loop of resistance band)

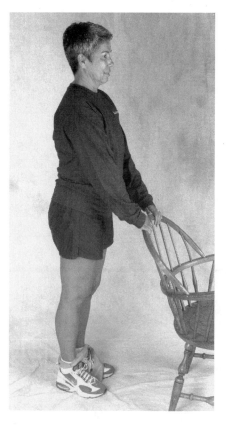

Stand with proper posture. Place both hands on the back of a sturdy chair. Loop the band around both ankles.

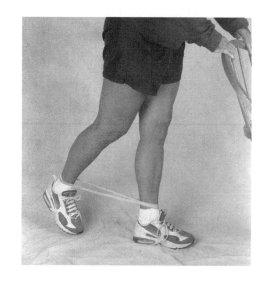

1
While keeping one foot firmly on the floor, tighten your buttocks and pull the band backward with your opposite foot.

2
Feel the muscles working in your hip and thigh.

3
Slowly return to the starting position. Repeat 10 times with each leg.

Outer Knee Press

Sit with proper posture and place your hands on the outside of your knees.

1

Push outward with your knees, resisting this motion with your hands.

2

Your legs will not move, but you will feel the muscles working in your thighs and buttocks.

3

Hold for 5 seconds.

4

Release. Repeat 10 times.

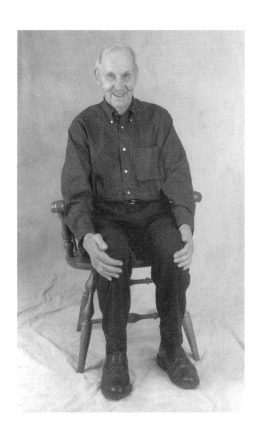

Inner Knee Press

Sit with proper posture and place your hands on the inside of your knees.

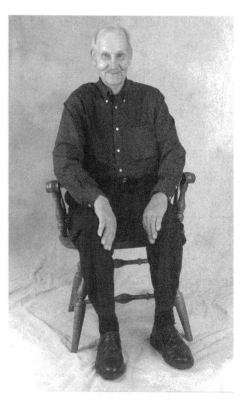

1
Push inward with your knees, resisting this motion with your hands.

2
Your legs will not move, but you will feel the muscles working in your thighs.

3
Hold for 5 seconds.

4
Release. Repeat 10 times.

Arm Curls
(use a length of resistance band)

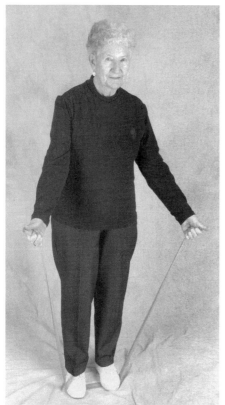

Stand on the band, grasping each end with your palms facing forward. Maintain proper posture.

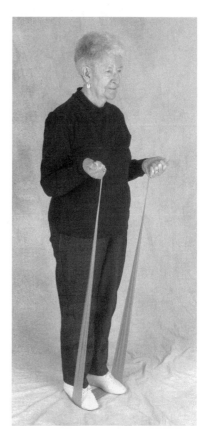

1
Keeping your elbows stationary and close to your body, bend your arms and bring your hands toward your shoulders, palms up. (Keep your upper body still.)

2
Feel the muscles working in your upper arms.

3
Slowly return to the starting position. Repeat 10 times.

"Cross Country" Skiing
(use a length of resistance band)

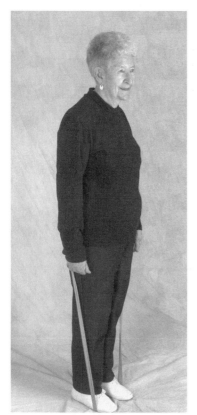

Stand on the band, grasping each end with your palms facing inward. Tighten your abdominal muscles and maintain proper posture.

1

Bring one arm forward and the other arm behind.

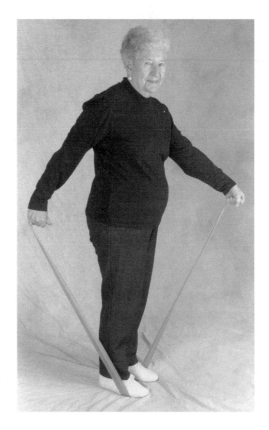

2

Now switch, bringing your other arm forward and the opposite arm behind.

3

Feel the muscles working in your shoulders. Repeat 10 times.

Wrist Curls—Palm Up
(use a length of resistance band)

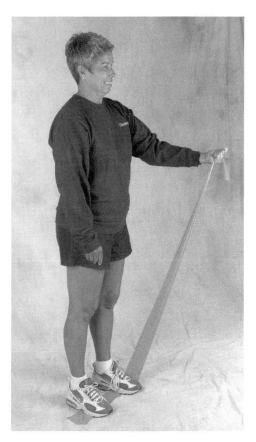

Stand on one end of the band and grasp the other end in one hand, palm up. Hold your forearm steady. Keep your elbow slightly bent and at your side throughout the exercise. Maintain proper posture.

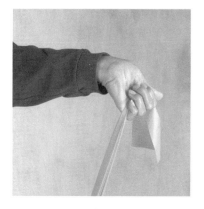

1
Slowly bend your wrist backward and down.

2
Slowly curl it up. Repeat 10 times with each wrist.

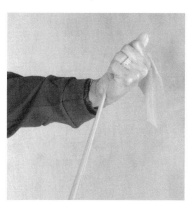

Wrist Curls—Palm Down
(use a length of resistance band)

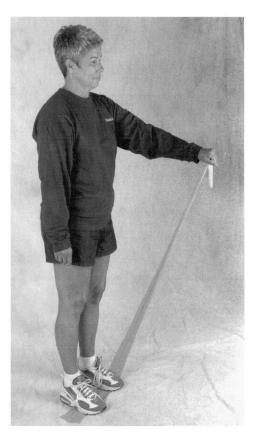

Stand on one end of the band and grasp the other end in one hand, palm down. Hold your forearm steady. Keep your elbow slightly bent and at your side throughout the exercise. Maintain proper posture.

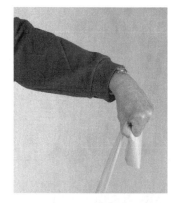

1

Slowly curl your wrist forward and down.

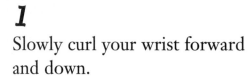

2

Slowly bend it up and back. Repeat 10 times with each wrist.

This completes your strengthening exercises. You are now ready to "warm down" with some stretching exercises.

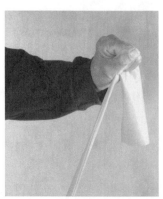

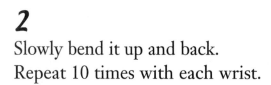

WARM-DOWN STRETCHING EXERCISES

A gentle stretching session is the perfect way to "warm down." Stretching also makes your joints and muscles more flexible. In fact, stretching has been shown to decrease many aches and pains associated with advancing age.

Ease into each stretch until you feel a gentle pull or tug along the muscle. Do not bounce. You should not feel pain. If you do, review the technique for the stretch and try again. If you still have pain, leave that particular stretch out of your routine.

Perform each stretch twice, holding for twenty seconds. Do all stretches while standing tall and straight, your ears aligned with your shoulders.

Neck Stretch

Stand with proper posture.

1

Tilt your head to the side, moving your ear toward your shoulder.

2

Feel the stretch along the side of your neck.

3

Hold for 20 seconds.

4

Return your head to an upright position. Do the stretch 2 times on each side.

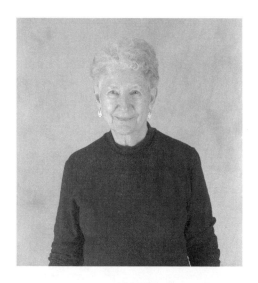 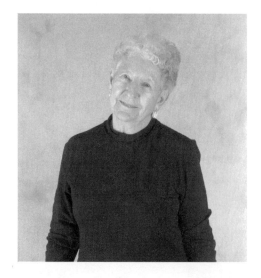

Shoulder Stretch–across the Body

Stand with proper posture. Bring one arm across your body, resting your hand on your shoulder.

1

Using your other hand, gently pull your elbow farther across your body.

2

Feel the stretch along the back of your shoulder.

3

Hold for 20 seconds.

4

Release the stretch briefly. Do the stretch 2 times with each arm.

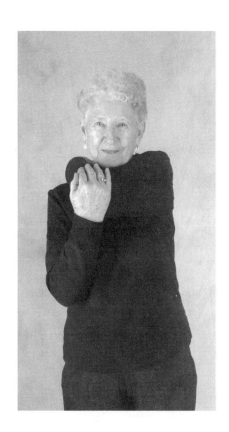

Wrist Stretch—Backward

Stand with proper posture. Extend one arm straight in front of you, elbow locked.

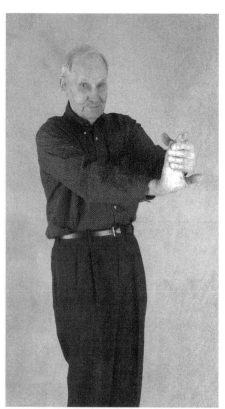

1

Using your other hand, gently pull your fingers back.

2

Hold for 20 seconds.

3

Release the stretch briefly. Do the stretch 2 times with each wrist.

Wrist Stretch—Forward

Stand with proper posture. Extend one arm straight in front of you, elbow locked.

1

Using your other hand, gently pull your fingers downward and back.

2

Hold for 20 seconds.

3

Release the stretch briefly. Do the stretch 2 times with each wrist.

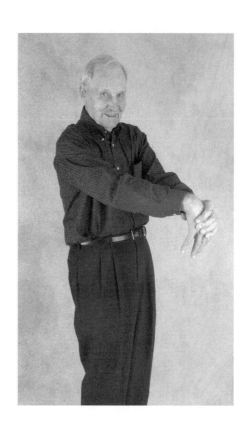

Calf Stretch

Stand with your hands on the back of a sturdy chair. Place one foot behind your body, keeping the leg straight. Maintain proper posture throughout the exercise.

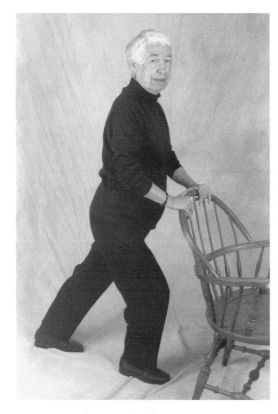

1

With your toes pointing straight ahead and your heels flat on the floor, gently lunge forward.

2

Feel the stretch in your calf.

3

Hold for 20 seconds.

4

Release the stretch briefly. Do the stretch 2 times with each leg.

Thigh Stretch

Stand with proper posture and place one hand on the back of a sturdy chair.

1

Grasp one foot and bring the heel to your buttocks; do not bend at the waist.

2

Feel the stretch along the front of your thigh.

3

Hold for 20 seconds.

4

Release the stretch briefly. Do the stretch 2 times with each leg.

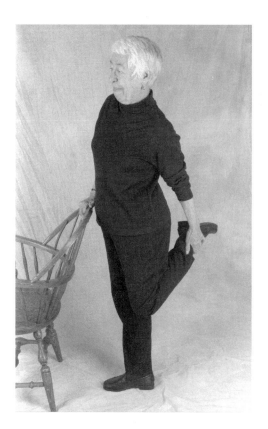

CONCLUSION

A diagnosis of osteoporosis does not mean you can no longer exercise. In fact, exercise, especially strength training, is an important part of slowing or reversing bone loss. When done safely, strength training can limit—and even help prevent— the disabling potential of osteoporosis.

Elizabeth Smith received degrees in athletic training and physical therapy from the University of Wisconsin, Madison. She supervises an outpatient clinic for Fairview Rehabilitation Services and provides care to a variety of patients. She specializes in evaluating and designing exercise programs for patients with osteoporosis and those predisposed to this condition. Elizabeth and her husband, Kevin, live in St. Paul.

Lorie A. Schleck is a physical therapist at Fairview Rehabilitation Services. She received her BS degree in physical therapy from the University of Minnesota and her MA degree in counseling psychology from St. Mary's University of Minnesota. Lorie and her husband, Jim, have a son, Ben, and a daughter, Kara.

6

Balance and Strength Training

Debbie Hanka, PT
Lorie A. Schleck, MA, PT

This program takes about 20 minutes.
Do it 3 to 5 times a week.

EQUIPMENT NEEDED:
  Comfortable, nonbinding clothing
  Athletic shoes with good arch support
  A stable, heavy chair that will not tip over, or the kitchen sink

---

Every year, one out of three people 65 or older suffers a fall. Some of these falls result in serious injury, even death. In fact, falls contribute to 40 percent of nursing home admissions. Studies show that 90 percent of all hip fractures are the result of a fall, and 20 percent of people who break a hip die within one year of the injury.

Falling is a serious threat to our health and independence. Each of us must think about fall prevention, especially if we've already fallen or if we're starting to feel off-balance.

Some of us are more at risk of falling than others. Risk factors include:

- Acute or chronic illness
- Four or more medications
- Low or high blood pressure
- Impaired vision or hearing
- Alcohol use
- Unsafe home
- Loss of muscle strength and flexibility
- Walking and balance problems

While certain risk factors are beyond our control—illness, medications, blood pressure—there are steps we can take to decrease our chances of falling.

PREVENTING FALLS

A fall can happen in less than a second, but its effects can last a lifetime. The time to take action is BEFORE a serious injury occurs. You can start right now by addressing two very important areas in your life: home safety and muscle strength.

Home Safety

Because most falls occur at or around the home, you can minimize your chances of falling by keeping your home safe and hazard-free. Use the following chart to identify and correct potential hazards in your home.

Hazard	Correction
A dark path from the bedroom to the bathroom.	Use night-lights to illuminate your path.
Nothing to hold on to when getting in and out of the tub or shower.	Install grab bars.
A slippery shower floor or bathtub.	Install nonskid strips or a nonslip mat.
Telephone, light, or television cords in walkways.	Reroute cords so they do not cross walkways.
Cluttered floors.	Remove clutter from walkways.
Getting up frequently at night to go to the bathroom.	Place a portable commode near your bed.
Reaching far from bed to get eyeglasses, the phone, or the light.	Place these items close to your bed.
Frayed corners or rolled-up edges on carpets or floor coverings.	Remove damaged floor coverings, or secure them with nails or double-sided tape.
Throw rugs in walkways.	Remove throw rugs, or secure them with double-sided tape.
Reaching up to pull cords for lights or ceiling fans.	Install longer cords, or link ceiling fans and lights to wall switches.
Unsafe stairways.	Stairways should be well-lit and have sturdy handrails on both sides.

Muscle Strength

Without exercise muscles become weak, which greatly increases your risk of falling. A balance and strength-training program will go a long way toward strong muscles, flexible joints, and improved balance, reducing your risk and perhaps preventing serious injury. Remember: "An ounce of prevention is worth a pound of cure."

THE PROGRAM

This program is designed to improve both balance and strength, critical factors in fall prevention. The exercises will require you to stand on one leg while moving the other. Over time, both your strength and balance will improve, and you will need less and less support.

Exercise Guidelines
- Wear comfortable, nonbinding clothing.
- Maintain proper body alignment: Stand tall and straight.
- Use an appropriate level of support throughout each exercise.
- Perform exercises slowly and smoothly.
- Do exercises in a pain-free range of motion.
- Do not progress too quickly.
- Begin with a warm-up session.

Safety Reminders
- Do not hold your breath while exercising.
- Stop immediately if you are short of breath.
- Stop immediately if you become fatigued.
- Exercises should not cause pain.

WARM-UP EXERCISES

The purpose of the warm-up is to increase blood flow to key muscle groups just before strength training. The warm-up takes four to five minutes. Any fairly vigorous activity can be substituted for this warm-up as long as it is done just before the strengthening exercises and it increases your heart rate slightly.

Gently and steadily perform the described movements for the designated time. When you are done, your heart rate should be slightly faster, and you should be breathing slightly harder. You should not feel fatigued. If you do, stop immediately.

Arm Swings

Steady yourself with one hand on the back of a sturdy chair, and stand with proper posture.

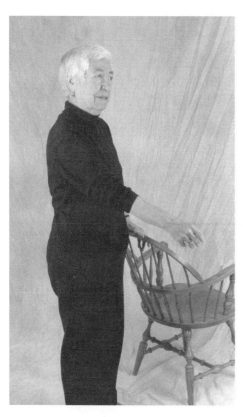

1

Swing one arm back and forth for 30 to 60 seconds.

2

Switch hands, then swing the other arm back and forth for 30 to 60 seconds.

Leg Swings

Stand with proper posture. Steady yourself with one
hand on the back of a sturdy chair and keep your
trunk still throughout the exercise.

1

Swing one leg back and forth for 60 seconds.

2

Swing your other leg back and forth for 60 seconds.

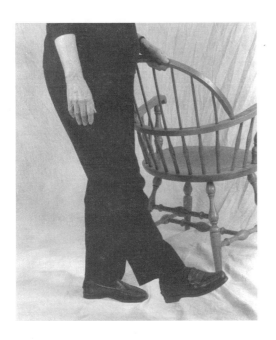
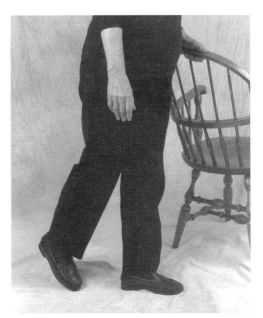

This completes your warm-up. You are now ready to start the
strength-training exercises.

STRENGTHENING AND STRETCHING EXERCISES

The following exercises will help you improve strength, flexibility, and balance. Use a kitchen sink or a stable, heavy chair (one that won't tip over) for support.

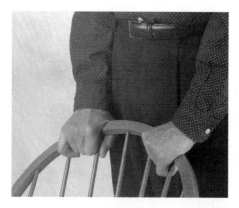

At first, do these exercises while grasping the sink or chair with both hands.

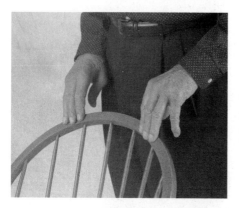

As your balance and strength improve, use fingertip support—place your fingertips lightly on the supporting surface.

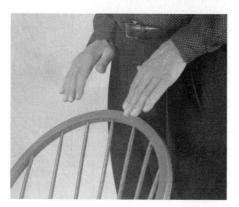

Finally, when you feel ready, do the exercises without holding on to anything. But stay close to a firm, supportive surface in case you become unsteady.

Side Leg Lifts

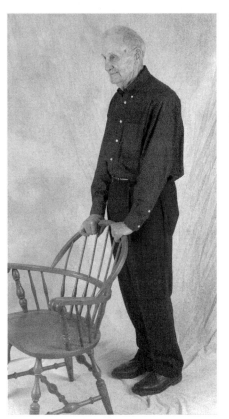

Stand with proper posture and place both hands on the kitchen sink or the back of a sturdy chair.

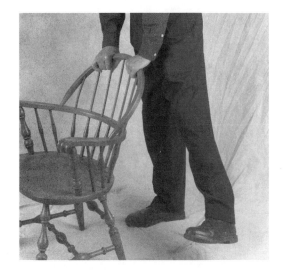

1

Tighten your buttocks and slowly lift one leg out to the side.

2

Feel the muscles working along the side of your hip.

3

Slowly lower your leg back to the floor. Repeat 10 times with each leg.

Backward Leg Lifts

Stand with proper posture and place both hands on the kitchen sink or the back of a sturdy chair.

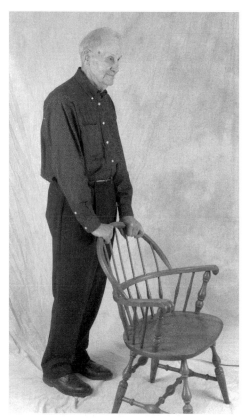

1
Lift one leg behind you, keeping your trunk upright and your leg straight.

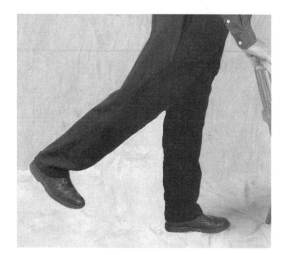

2
Feel the muscles working in your buttocks and in the back of your thigh.

3
Slowly lower your leg back to the floor. Repeat 10 times with each leg.

Leg Curls

Stand with proper posture and place both hands on the kitchen sink or the back of a sturdy chair.

1

Bend one knee and lift your lower leg off the ground.

2

Feel the muscles working in the back of your thigh.

3

Slowly lower your leg back to the floor. Repeat 10 times with each leg.

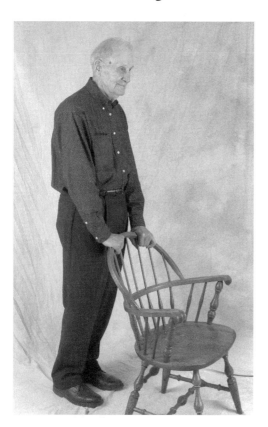

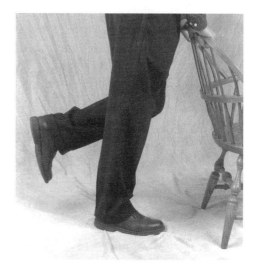

Thigh Lifts

Standing sideways with proper posture, place one
hand on the kitchen sink or the back of a sturdy chair.

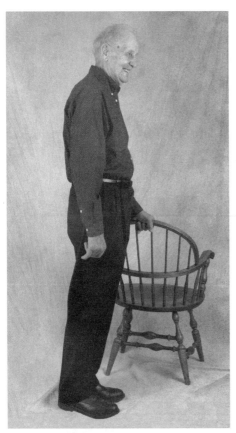

1

Bring one knee up to hip level.

2

Feel the muscles working along the
front of your thigh.

3

Slowly lower your foot back to
the floor. Repeat 10 times with
each leg.

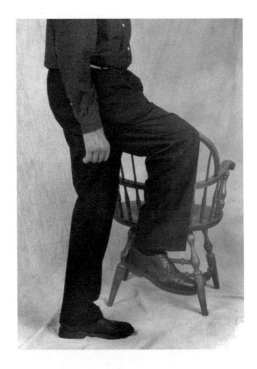

Thigh Stretch

Stand with proper posture and place one hand on the kitchen sink or the back of a sturdy chair.

1

Grasp one foot and bring the heel to your buttocks; do not bend at the waist.

2

Feel the stretch along the front of your thigh.

3

Hold for 20 seconds.

4

Release the stretch briefly. Do this stretch 2 times with each leg.

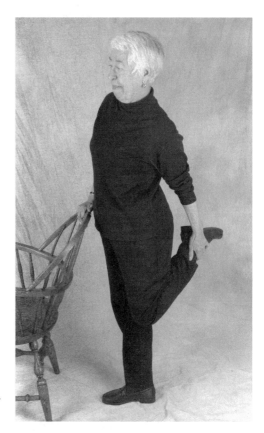

Toe Lifts

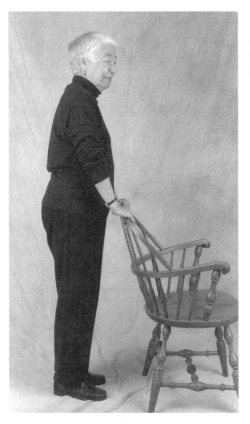

Stand with proper posture and place both hands on the kitchen sink or the back of a sturdy chair.

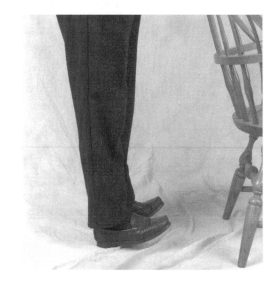

1
Raise the balls of your feet off the floor.

2
Feel the muscles working in your shins.

3
Slowly lower the balls of your feet back to the floor. Repeat 10 times.

Heel Lifts

Stand with proper posture and place both hands on the kitchen sink or the back of a sturdy chair.

1

Raise both heels off the floor.

2

Feel the muscles working in your calves.

3

Slowly lower your heels to the ground. Repeat 10 times.

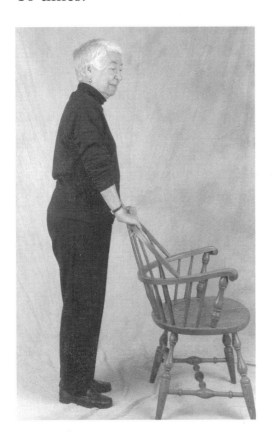

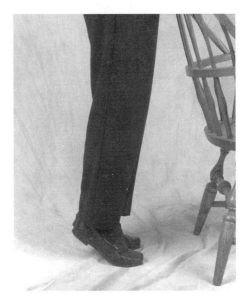

Calf Stretch

Stand with both hands on the kitchen sink or the back of a sturdy chair. Place one foot behind your body, keeping the leg straight. Maintain proper posture throughout the exercise.

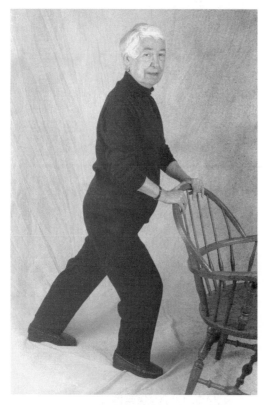

1
With your toes pointing straight ahead and your heels flat on the floor, gently lunge forward.

2
Feel the stretch in your calf.

3
Hold for 20 seconds.

4
Release the stretch briefly. Do the stretch 2 times with each leg.

Shoulder Rolls

Stand near the kitchen sink or a sturdy chair. If you feel unsteady, grasp the sink or chair for support. Maintain proper posture throughout the exercise.

1

Roll both shoulders backward, making a circle. Repeat 10 times.

2

Roll your shoulders forward, making a circle. Repeat 10 times.

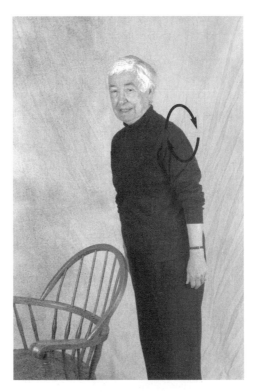

This completes your strengthening and stretching exercises.

Conclusion

No one should risk losing everything because of one bad fall. If you experience balance problems or muscle weakness, if you have fallen even once, use the exercises and fall prevention tips in this chapter. Protect your health, your mobility, and your independence. Make fall prevention a priority.

Debbie Hanka is the program coordinator for Preventing Falls in Older Adults at Fairview Ridges Hospital. She received her BS degree in physical therapy from the University of Minnesota. Debbie and her husband, Greg, have three children, Emily, Ben, and Ian.

Lorie A. Schleck is a physical therapist at Fairview Rehabilitation Services. She received her BS degree in physical therapy from the University of Minnesota and her MA degree in counseling psychology from St. Mary's University of Minnesota. Lorie and her husband, Jim, have a son, Ben, and a daughter, Kara.

7

Strength Training for Golfers

Karen Oelschlaeger, PT
Lorie A. Schleck, MA, PT

This programs takes 30 to 40 minutes.
Do it 2 to 3 times a week.
A 48-hour break is recommended between each session.
Do the warm-down stretching exercises every day.

EQUIPMENT NEEDED:
  Stable, heavy chair that will not tip over
  Chair with armrests
  Stool
  Railing, kitchen sink, or heavy piece of furniture
  Length of resistance band (3 to 4 feet)
  Loop of resistance band
  Door
  Rolled-up towel
  Golf club
  Small cuff weights (optional)
  Athletic shoes with good arch support

Golf is a popular activity among older adults. But to play well, avoid injury, and enjoy the game, golfers require a certain level of strength and flexibility. This means that regular strength-training and stretching exercises are essential. Without them, our balance, timing, and coordination suffer. We become prone to injury, and by age 65, we could lose over 20 percent of the strength we had when we were 25.

Older adults who play golf regularly need to maintain their fitness. In his book *Physical Golf*, Neil Wolkodoff outlines the following fitness recommendations for older golfers:

- Exercise regularly.
- Increase warm-up time before and warm-down time after golfing to make up for reduced circulation.
- Perform stretching exercises daily.
- Do aerobic conditioning.
- Engage in sports off-season to improve coordination.
- Participate in a golf-specific strength-training program twice a week.

If you follow these guidelines—and take advantage of the strength-training exercises in this chapter—you'll be on your way to golfing fitness in no time.

THE PROGRAM

Strength Training for Golfers consists of a warm-up session, strengthening exercises, and warm-down stretching exercises. You may want to meet with a physical therapist or other health-care professional before beginning this program. A trained professional can help make sure you are exercising properly.

Exercise Guidelines
- Wear comfortable, nonbinding clothing.
- Maintain proper body alignment:
  - For standing exercises, stand tall and straight.
  - For sitting exercises, sit tall with your feet firmly on the floor.
- Perform each exercise slowly and smoothly.
- Do each exercise in a pain-free range of motion.
- Do not increase resistance too quickly.
- Begin with a warm-up session.
- End with the warm-down stretching exercises.

Safety Reminders
- Do not hold your breath while exercising.
- Stop immediately if you are short of breath.
- Stop immediately if you become fatigued.
- Exercises should not cause pain.

WARM-UP EXERCISES

The purpose of the warm-up is to increase blood flow to key muscle groups just before strength training. The warm-up takes four to five minutes. Any fairly vigorous activity can be substituted for this warm-up as long as it is done just before the strengthening exercises and it increases your heart rate slightly.

Gently and steadily perform the described movements for the designated time. When you are done, your heart rate should be slightly faster, and you should be breathing slightly harder. You should not feel fatigued. If you do, stop immediately.

Arm Swings

Stand with proper posture.

1

Swing both arms, alternating one forward and one backward, for 60 seconds.

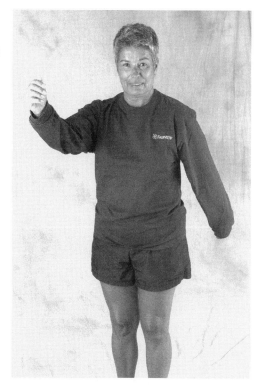

Leg Swings

Stand with proper posture. Steady yourself with one hand on the back of a sturdy chair and keep your trunk still throughout the exercise.

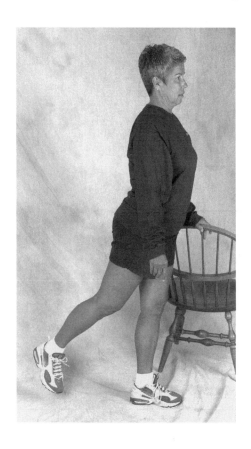 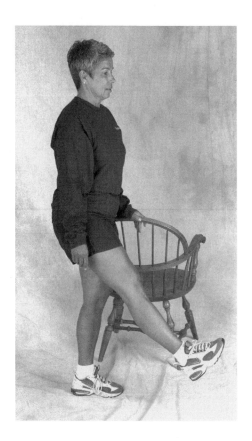

1

Swing one leg back and forth for 60 seconds.

2

Swing your other leg back and forth for 60 seconds.

This completes your warm-up. You are now ready to start the strength-training exercises.

STRENGTHENING EXERCISES

Strength Training for Golfers includes thirteen exercises for
key muscle groups in your arms, legs, and trunk. If an exercise
causes pain, limit your range of motion during that exercise.
For example, if it hurts to straighten your leg, don't straighten
it all the way. If you still have pain while limiting the motion,
do not do the exercise.

Some exercises call for a length of resistance band. Others
call for a loop of band. To make a loop, tie the ends of the
band together.

For exercises without a Thera-Band resistance band:
- Begin with 10 repetitions.
- As the exercises get easier, progress to 12 and then
  to 15 repetitions.
- Next, progress to two sets of 10, then 12, then
  15 repetitions.
- Finally, if able, progress to three sets of 10, then 12,
  then 15 repetitions.

For exercises with a Thera-Band resistance band:
- Begin with 10 repetitions.
- As the exercises get easier, progress to 12 and then
  to 15 repetitions.
- Next, move to a higher level band and do 10, then 12,
  then 15 repetitions.
- After you reach your ideal level of resistance, do two
  sets of 10, then 12, then 15.
- Finally, if able, progress to three sets of 10, then 12,
  then 15 repetitions.

Arm Roll-Outs
(use a resistance band and a rolled-up towel)

This exercise improves your ability to pull a club back and swing.

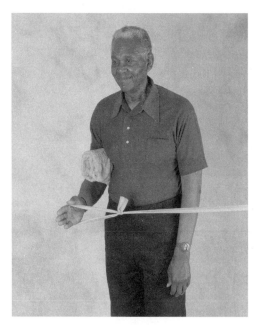

Stand sideways next to a door. Tie a knot in one end of the band and close it in the door at waist level. Tie a loop in the other end and place it around the wrist farthest from the door. Bend your arm 90 degrees and tuck a towel under your elbow for support. Maintain proper posture throughout the exercise.

1

Roll your forearm out from your body, pulling on the band as you do so. (Keep your elbow bent at a 90-degree angle.)

2

Feel the muscles working in your shoulder.

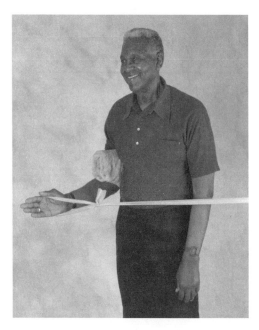

3

Slowly return to the starting position. Repeat 10 times with each arm.

Arm Roll-Ins
(use a resistance band and a rolled-up towel)

This exercise improves your ability to pull a club back and swing.

Stand sideways next to a door. Tie a knot in one end of the band and close it in the door at waist level. Tie a loop in the other end and place it around the wrist nearest the door. Bend your arm 90 degrees and tuck a towel beneath your elbow for support. Maintain proper posture throughout the exercise.

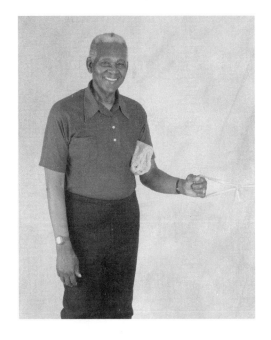

1

Pull the band in toward your body.

2

Feel the muscles working in your shoulder.

3

Slowly return to the starting position. Repeat 10 times with each arm.

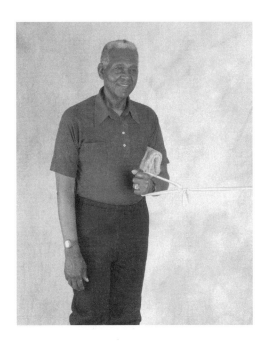

Pull-Downs
(use a length of resistance band)

This exercise aids stability and control during your golf swing.

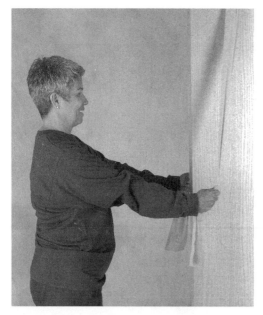

Drape the band over the top of an open door (4 to 6 inches from the door's edge, so it doesn't slip). Grasp each end, keeping your arms straight.

1

Squeezing your shoulder blades together, pull the band down to your thighs. (Keep your elbows close to your body.)

2

Feel the muscles working in your upper back and shoulders.

3

Slowly return to the starting position. Repeat 10 times.

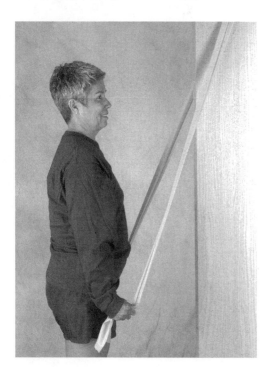

Wrist Curls—Palm Up
(use a length of resistance band)

This exercise helps you deliver more force when your club hits the ball.

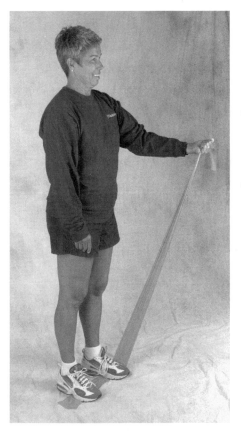

Stand on one end of the band and grasp the other end in one hand, palm up. Hold your forearm steady. Keep your elbow slightly bent and at your side throughout the exercise. Maintain proper posture.

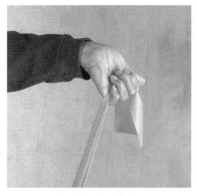

1
Slowly bend your wrist backward and down.

2
Slowly curl it up. Repeat 10 times with each wrist.

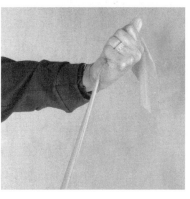

Wrist Curls—Palm Down
(use a length of resistance band)

This exercise helps you deliver more force when your club hits the ball.

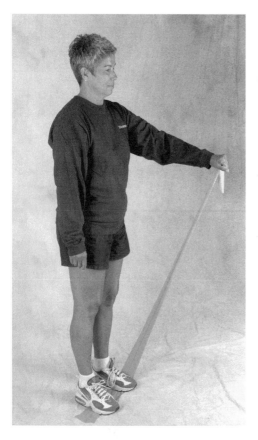

Stand on one end of the band and grasp the other end in one hand, palm down. Hold your forearm steady. Keep your elbow slightly bent and at your side throughout the exercise. Maintain proper posture.

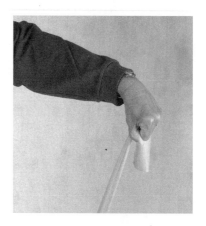

1
Slowly curl your wrist forward and down.

2
Slowly bend it up and back. Repeat 10 times with each wrist.

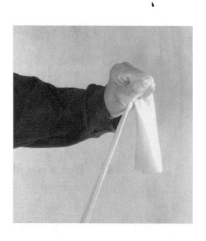

Wrist Tips
(use a golf club)

This exercise helps you develop a more powerful swing.

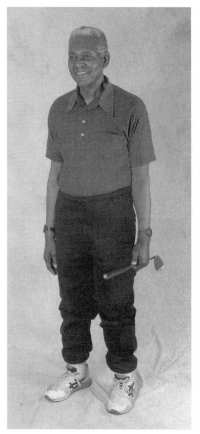

With your arm relaxed and at your side, hold a golf club in your hand (handle forward), grasping it in the center.

1

Tip your wrist so the handle of the golf club points toward the floor.

2

Feel the muscles working in your wrist and forearm.

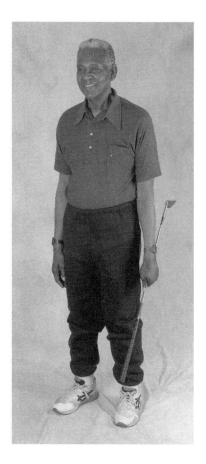

3

Slowly return to the starting position. Repeat 10 times with each wrist.

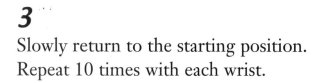

Half-Squat

This exercise improves leg strength for a proper golfing stance.

Stand with proper posture and set your feet shoulder-width apart. Hold on to something firm at about waist height, like a railing, a heavy piece of furniture, the kitchen sink, or another person.

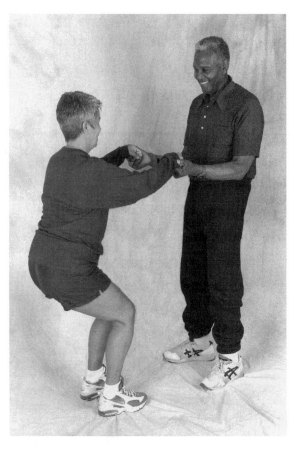

1
Bend your knees.

2
Slowly lower your body as if you were sitting down into a chair.

3
When you're partway down (about a quarter of the way), pause briefly.

4
Slowly return to the starting position, pushing up through your heels as you do so.

5
Throughout the movement, concentrate on using the muscles along the front of your thighs and your buttocks. Repeat 10 times.

Backward Leg Pulls
(use a loop of resistance band)

This exercise improves leg strength needed for a proper golfing stance and for bending down to retrieve your ball.

Stand with proper posture. Place both hands on the back of a sturdy chair. Loop the band around your ankles.

1
While keeping one foot firmly on the floor, tighten the buttocks and pull the band backward with your opposite foot.

2
Feel the muscles working in your hip and thigh.

3
Slowly return to the starting position. Repeat 10 times with each leg.

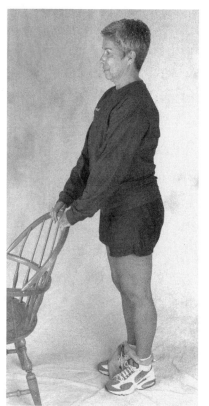

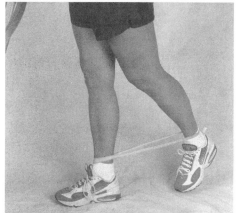

Side Leg Lifts
(use a loop of resistance band)

This exercise helps you develop a powerful swing and the stability needed for a proper golfing stance.

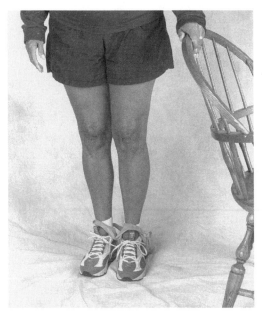

Stand sideways, feet together, with one hand on the back of a sturdy chair. Loop the band around both ankles. Keep the foot nearest the chair firmly on the floor, with the knee slightly bent. Maintain proper posture throughout the exercise.

1
Tighten your buttocks and slowly pull the band out to the side. (Keep your feet pointed straight ahead.)

2
Feel the muscles working along the outside of your hip and thigh.

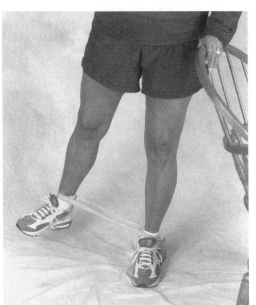

3
Slowly return your leg to the starting position. Repeat 10 times with each leg.

Abdominal Press

This exercise strengthens your back, protecting it from injury.

Lie flat on the floor, face up, with your knees bent. Place your hands on your stomach.

1

Tighten your stomach muscles while flattening your back against the floor.

2

Feel with your hands as your stomach muscles tighten.

3

Hold for 5 seconds.

4

Release. Repeat 10 times.

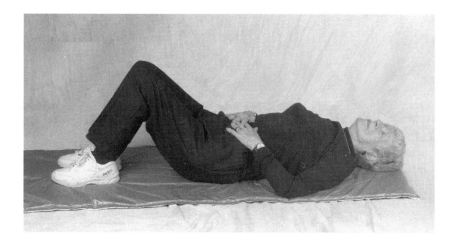

Arm Lifts

This exercise helps with trunk stability and coordination.

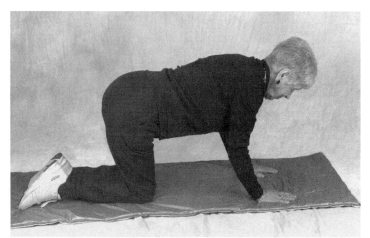

Get on your hands and knees. Keep your spine straight throughout this exercise—do not allow your back to sag or become rounded.

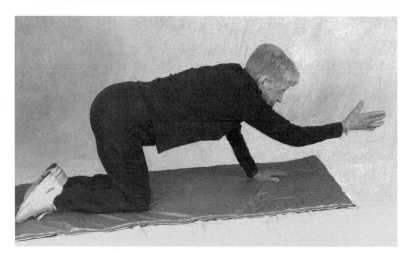

1
Tighten your abdominal muscles.

2
Lift one arm in front of you, pointing your thumb toward the ceiling.

3
Lower your arm to the floor. Lift the other arm in front of you, pointing your thumb toward the ceiling. Repeat 10 times.

As this exercise gets easier, do two or three sets, or add cuff weights for resistance.

Leg Lifts

This exercise helps with trunk stability and coordination.

Get on your hands and knees. Keep the spine straight—do not allow your lower back to sag during the exercise.

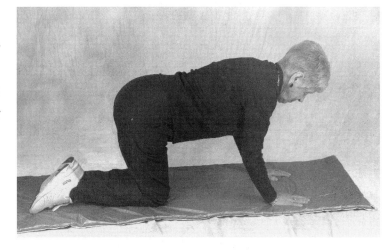

1
Tighten your abdominal muscles and keep your trunk still.

2
Lift one leg behind you.

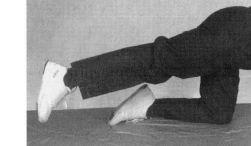

3
Lower your leg to the floor, then lift the other leg behind you. Repeat 10 times.

As this exercise gets easier, do two or three sets, or add cuff weights for resistance.

When arm lifts and leg lifts become too easy, even with resistance, go on to the next exercise—arm and leg lifts.

Arm and Leg Lifts

This exercise helps with trunk stability and coordination. Do this exercise only after the arm lifts and leg lifts become too easy.

Get on your hands and knees. Keep your spine straight—do not allow your lower back to sag during this exercise.

1
Tighten your abdominal muscles.

2
Simultaneously lift one arm and the opposite leg.

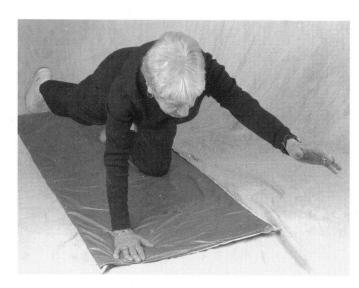

3
Return to the starting position.

4
Simultaneously lift the other arm and opposite leg. Repeat 10 times.

This completes your strengthening exercises. You are now ready to "warm down" with some stretching exercises.

WARM-DOWN STRETCHING EXERCISES

A gentle stretching session is the perfect way to "warm down." Stretching also makes your joints and muscles more flexible. In fact, stretching has been shown to decrease many aches and pains associated with advancing age.

Ease into each stretch until you feel a gentle pull or tug along the muscle. Do not bounce. You should not feel pain. If you do, review the technique for the stretch and try again. If you still have pain, leave that particular stretch out of your routine.

Do all stretches while standing or sitting tall and straight, your ears aligned with your shoulders.

Neck Rotation

Stand with proper posture.

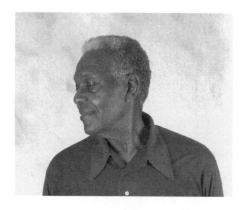

1

Slowly turn your head to look over one shoulder. Do not hold the stretch.

2

Return to the starting position.

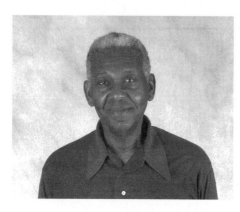

3

Slowly turn your head to look over your other shoulder. Do not hold the stretch.

4

Return to the starting position. Repeat 5 times.

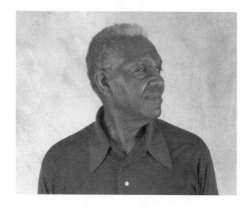

Wrist Stretch–Backward

Stand with proper posture. Extend one arm straight
in front of you, elbow locked.

1

Using your other hand, gently pull
your fingers back.

2

Hold for 20 seconds.

3

Release the stretch briefly. Do the
stretch 2 times with each wrist.

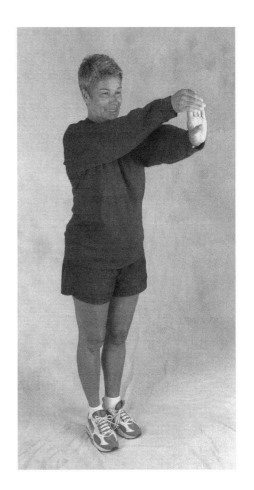

Wrist Stretch–Forward

Stand with proper posture. Extend one arm straight in front of you, elbow locked.

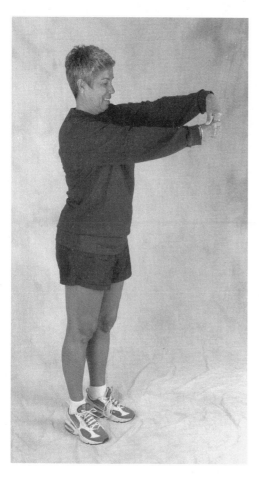

1

Using your other hand, gently pull your fingers downward and back.

2

Hold for 20 seconds.

3

Release the stretch briefly. Do the stretch 2 times with each wrist.

Shoulder Stretch—across the Body

Stand with proper posture. Bring one arm across your body, resting your hand on your shoulder.

1

Using your other hand, gently pull your elbow farther across your body.

2

Feel the stretch along the back of your shoulder.

3

Hold for 20 seconds.

4

Release the stretch briefly. Do the stretch 2 times with each arm.

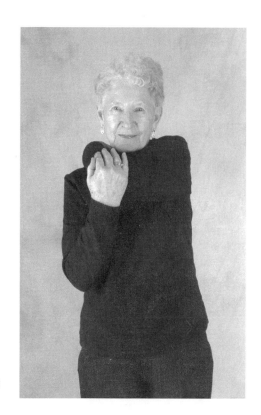

Chest Stretch
(use a golf club)

Stand or sit with proper posture. Hold a golf club over your head in both hands, palms facing forward.

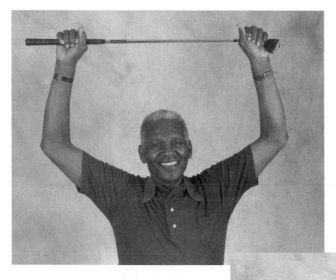

1
Pull your arms down, bringing the club behind your head.

2
Feel the stretch in your chest and shoulders. Hold for 20 seconds.

3
Return to the starting position. Repeat.

Trunk Rotation
(use a chair with armrests)

Sit with proper posture.

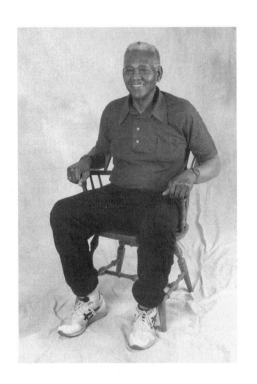

1

Twist your upper body to the left, using the armrests for support.

2

Hold for 5 seconds, feeling the stretch in your back and hips.

3

Slowly return to the starting position.

4

Twist your upper body to the right.

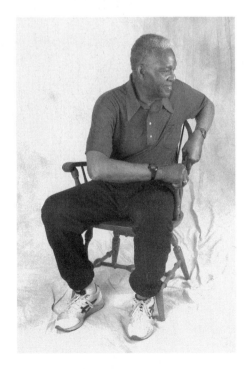

5

Hold for 5 seconds.

6

Slowly return to the starting position. Repeat 10 times.

Calf Stretch

Stand with your hands on the back of a sturdy chair. Place one foot behind your body with both knees bent. Maintain proper posture throughout the exercise.

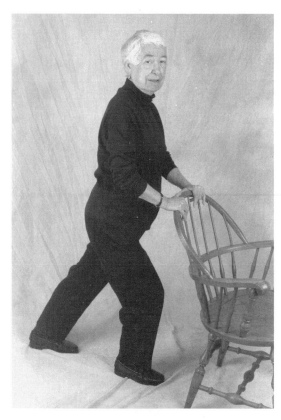

1
With your toes pointing straight ahead and your heels flat on the floor, gently lunge forward.

2
Feel the stretch in your calf.

3
Hold for 20 seconds.

4
Release the stretch briefly. Do the stretch 2 times with each leg.

Hamstring Stretch

Stand with proper posture and set one foot on the seat of a chair or stool.

1

Keeping your back straight, lean forward at your waist, being careful not to stretch too far and lose proper form.

2

Feel the gentle stretch along the back of your thigh.

3

Hold for 20 seconds.

4

Release the stretch briefly. Do the stretch 2 times with each leg.

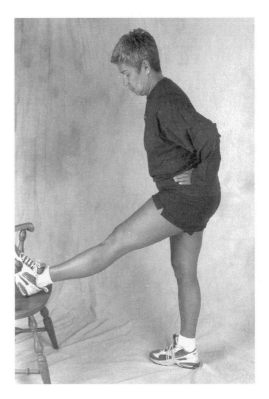

Thigh Stretch

Stand with proper posture and place one hand on the back of a sturdy chair.

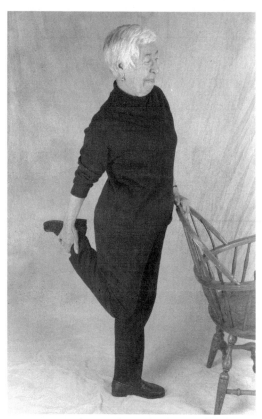

1

Grasp one foot and bring the heel to your buttocks; do not bend at the waist.

2

Feel the stretch along the front of your thigh.

3

Hold for 20 seconds.

4

Release the stretch briefly. Do the stretch 2 times with each leg.

Knee Press

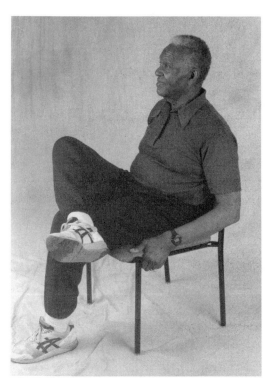

Sit with proper posture. Place your ankle on the opposite knee.

1

Place one hand on your knee, gently pressing the knee toward the floor.

2

Hold for 20 seconds, feeling the stretch along your thigh.

3

Release the stretch briefly. Repeat 2 times with each leg.

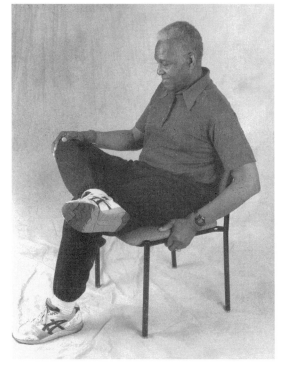

Outer Knee Press

Stand with proper posture. Place one foot flat on a chair with your hand on your knee.

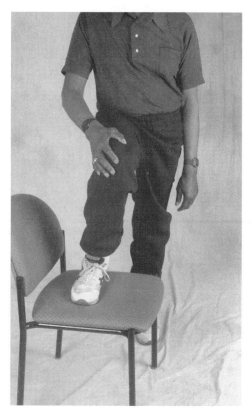

1

Use your hand to press the knee inward.

2

Hold for 20 seconds. Feel the stretch along your thigh.

3

Release. Do the exercise 2 times with each leg.

CONCLUSION

Many people enjoy golfing well into older age. This strength-training program can help minimize the tendency of aging muscles to become weaker and tighter, giving you the strength and flexibility you need to keep playing the game you love.

Karen Oelschlaeger is a physical therapist with Fairview Rehabilitation Services, where she works in sports medicine. She is involved with The Golf Program, which specializes in rehabilitating injured golfers. Ms. Oelschlaeger received a BA degree from Augustana College in Sioux Falls, South Dakota, and her physical therapy degree from the University of Minnesota. Karen and her husband, Terry Ruane, live in St. Louis Park, Minnesota.

Lorie A. Schleck is a physical therapist at Fairview Rehabilitation Services. She received her BS degree in physical therapy from the University of Minnesota and her MA degree in counseling psychology from St. Mary's University of Minnesota. Lorie and her husband, Jim, have a son, Ben, and a daughter, Kara.

8

Strength Training in the Pool

Lorie A. Schleck, MA, PT

Once you're in the pool, this program takes 20 to 30 minutes.
Do it 2 to 3 times each week.
A 48-hour break is recommended between each session.

EQUIPMENT NEEDED:
   Swimsuit
   Water socks

For many of us, the swimming pool is an ideal place for strength training. The water provides the resistance we need to work our muscles, so there's no need for weights or exercise bands. And because the resistance varies according to our ability, there's less chance of injury.

TIPS FOR STRENGTH TRAINING IN THE POOL

The water temperature should be between 82 and 86 degrees Fahrenheit. This will ensure a comfortable and effective work-out. Water that is too cold will cause muscles to tighten up, and this can lead to injury. On the other hand, water that is too warm may cause early fatigue.

Ideally, the water should reach your mid-chest. If the water is too shallow, you can bend your knees or stand with your legs apart to get more of your body under water.

Pool bottoms can be slippery, and so can the walk between the shower and the pool. Also, if the pool bottom is textured or tiled, it can scrape the soles of your feet. Consider buying a pair of water socks, which have rubber soles to protect your feet and prevent slipping. Water socks are sold at most discount or department stores.

For safety reasons, no one should ever swim alone. Be certain that someone is nearby in case a medical emergency occurs.

THE PROGRAM

Strength Training in the Pool consists of a warm-up session, strengthening exercises, and warm-down stretching exercises. You may want to meet with a physical therapist or other health-care professional before beginning this program. A trained professional can help make sure you are exercising properly.

Exercise Guidelines
- Maintain proper body alignment: Stand tall and straight.
- Perform each exercise slowly and smoothly.
- Do each exercise in a pain-free range of motion.
- Do not increase resistance too quickly.
- Begin with a warm-up session.
- End with the warm-down stretching exercises.

Safety Reminders
- Never exercise in the pool alone.
- Wear water socks to prevent slipping.
- Do not hold your breath while exercising.
- Stop immediately if you are short of breath.
- Stop immediately if you become fatigued.
- Exercises should not cause pain.

WARM-UP EXERCISES

Before strength training in the pool, always warm up to prepare your muscles for exercise. Do your warm-up in water that reaches between your waist and mid-chest. When you're done with the warm-up, your breathing should be slightly faster.

Walking or Jogging

Start by simply walking or jogging, either in place or across the pool, for 1 to 2 minutes. Be sure to move your arms as well as your legs.

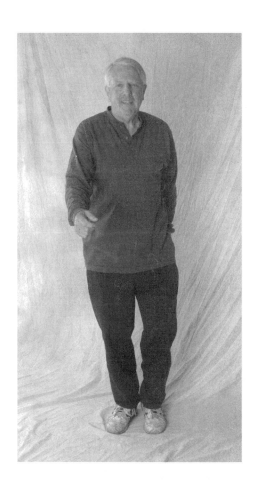

Sidestepping

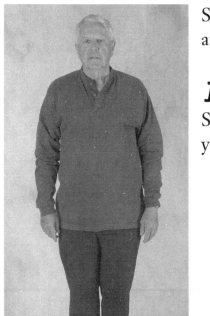

Stand with proper posture, your hands
at your sides.

1

Step one leg out to the side and raise
your arms to shoulder level.

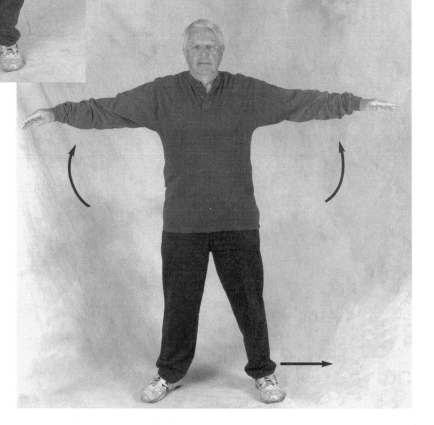

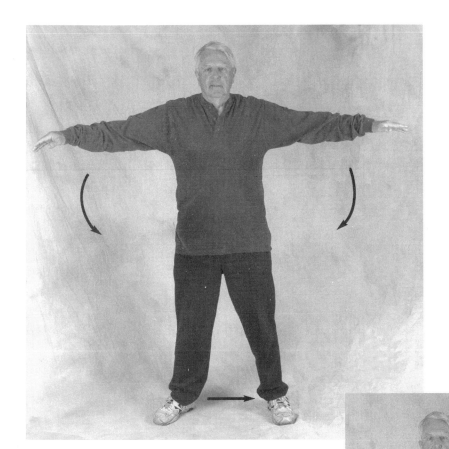

2

Bring the other leg in (so your feet are together) while lowering your arms to your sides.

3

Keep sidestepping back and forth for 60 seconds, or in the same direction for 30 seconds (be sure to repeat in the opposite direction).

Marching

Bringing your knees up to hip level, march either in place or across the pool for 60 seconds. Move each arm naturally with the opposite leg.

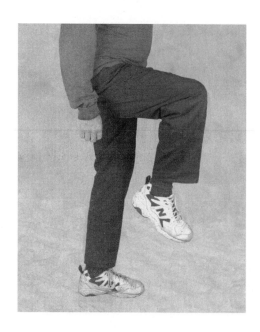

Walking or Jogging (Repeat)

Walk or jog, either in place or across the pool, for 1 to 2 minutes. Be sure to move your arms as well as your legs.

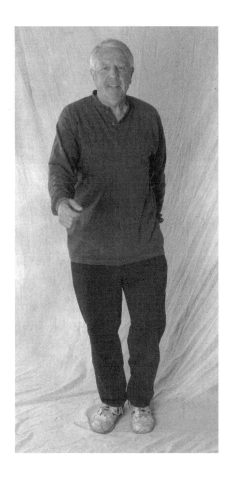

This completes your warm-up. You are now ready to start strength-training exercises.

STRENGTHENING EXERCISES

When strength training in the pool, you will do each exercise while standing up to your mid-chest in water. You'll move your limbs through the water to create resistance. The faster you move, the greater the resistance. You'll know you're building strength when your muscles are tired after completing a set of repetitions. If your muscles are not tired after a given exercise, try moving your limbs faster or adding more repetitions.

If any exercise causes pain, limit your range of motion during that exercise. For example, if it hurts to straighten your leg, don't straighten it all the way. If you still have pain while limiting the motion, do not do the exercise.

For each exercise:
- Begin with 10 repetitions.
- As the exercises get easier, progress to 12 and then to 15 repetitions.
- Next, progress to two sets of 10, then 12, then 15 repetitions.
- Finally, if able, progress to three sets of 10, then 12, then 15 repetitions.

Arm Swings

Stand with proper posture.

1

Bring one arm forward and the other arm backward, keeping your elbows locked.

2

Stop just below the surface of the water and switch directions, bringing your opposite arm forward and the other arm backward.

3

Feel the muscles working in your shoulders and upper arms. Repeat 10 times.

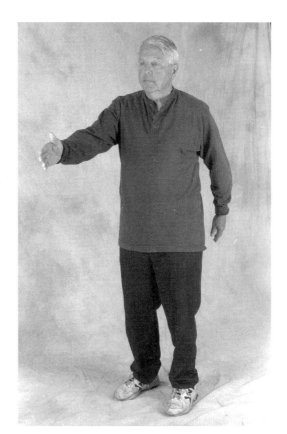

Use the placement of your hands to increase or decrease the resistance. If your palms face inward, they are more streamlined, creating less resistance. If your palms are turned to face behind you, the surface area is increased, creating more resistance. Choose a position that leaves your shoulder muscles slightly tired after 10 repetitions.

Forearm Pumps

Stand with proper posture, arms at your sides, palms forward.

1

Bend your arms, bringing your hands up to your shoulders.

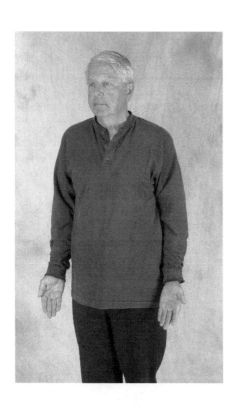
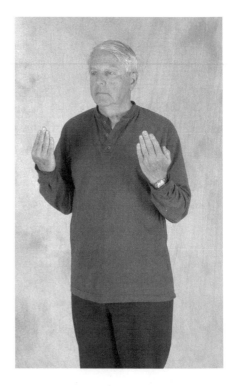

2

Turn your hands over so your palms face forward.
Push down, straightening your arms.

3

Feel the muscles working in your upper arms. Repeat
10 times.

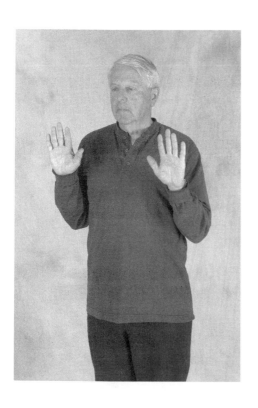
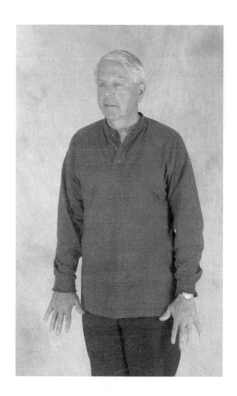

Forward Arm Swings

Stand with proper posture. Extend your arms straight out to the sides, palms facing forward.

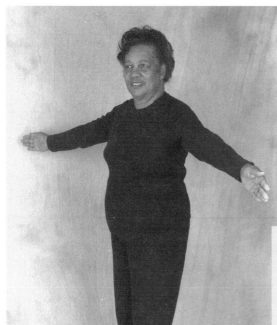

1

Keeping your elbows locked, pull your hands together.

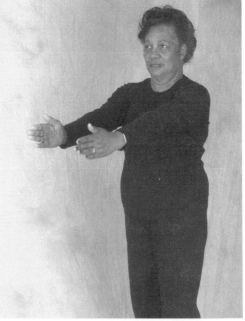

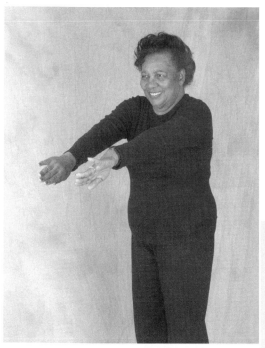

2

After your hands meet in front, turn your hands so your palms face outward.

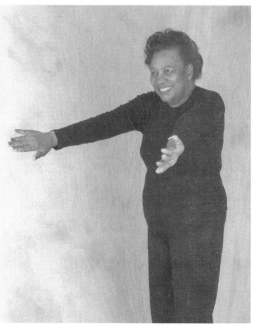

3

Keeping your elbows locked, push your hands back out to the sides.

4

Feel the muscles working in your shoulders and upper arms. Repeat 10 times.

Arms Lifts

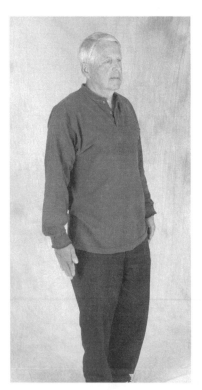

Stand with proper posture, hands at your sides, palms facing inward.

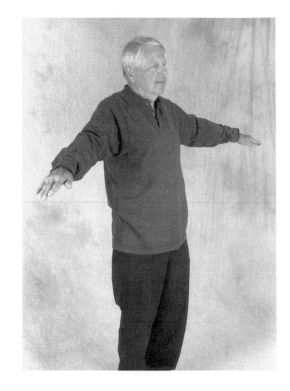

1
Lift your arms out to the sides, keeping your elbows locked.

2
Stop just below the water's surface, then pull your arms back to the starting position.

3
Feel the muscles working in your arms. Repeat 10 times.

Legs Swings

Stand sideways at the edge of the pool, holding on to the edge for balance. Maintain proper posture throughout the exercise; do not allow your trunk to move forward or backward.

1

Lift one foot off the ground and swing your leg backward.

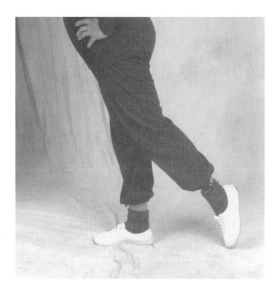

2

Swing the leg forward.

3

Feel the muscles working along your thigh and buttocks.
Repeat 10 times with each leg.

Side Legs Lifts

Stand sideways at the edge of the pool, holding on to the edge with one hand. Maintain proper posture throughout the exercise.

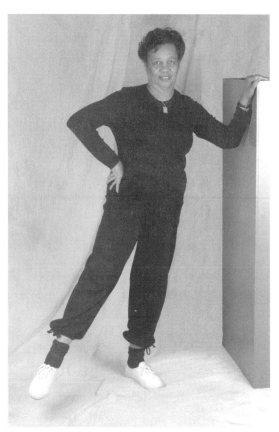

1

Lift your leg out to the side.

2

Return to the starting position.

3

Feel the muscles working in your thigh and buttocks. Repeat 10 times with each leg.

Lower Leg "Kicks"

Stand sideways at the edge of the pool, holding on to the edge with one hand. Lift your thigh up to hip level, bending the knee at a 90-degree angle.

1

Point your toes, keep your upper leg stationary, and straighten your lower leg.

2

Return to the starting position.

3

Feel the muscles working in your thigh and knee. Repeat 10 times with each leg.

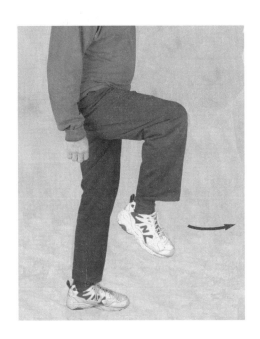

This completes your strengthening exercises. You are now ready to "warm down" with some stretching exercises.

WARM-DOWN STRETCHING EXERCISES

A gentle stretching session is the perfect way to "warm down." Stretching also makes your joints and muscles more flexible. In fact, stretching has been shown to decrease many aches and pains associated with advancing age.

Ease into each stretch until you feel a gentle pull or tug along the muscle. Do not bounce. You should not feel pain. If you do, review the technique for the stretch and try again. If you still have pain, leave that particular stretch out of your routine.

Perform each stretch twice, holding for twenty seconds. Do all stretches while standing tall and straight, your ears aligned with your shoulders.

Neck Stretch

Stand with proper posture.

1

Tilt your head to the side, moving your ear toward your shoulder.

2

Feel the stretch along the side of your neck.

3

Hold for 20 seconds.

4

Return your head to an upright position. Do the stretch 2 times on each side.

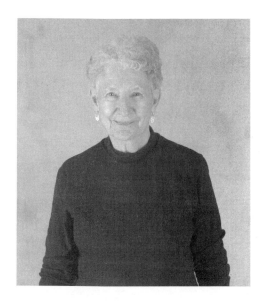 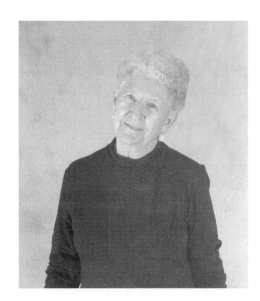

Shoulder Stretch—over the Head

Stand with proper posture. Place one hand at the back of your neck, pointing your elbow in the air.

1

Using your other hand, gently pull your elbow toward the middle of your back.

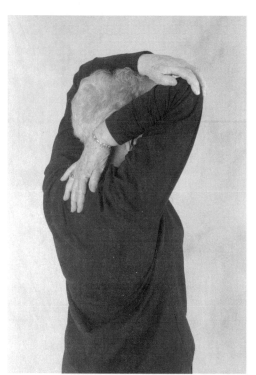

2

Feel the stretch along your shoulder.

3

Hold for 20 seconds.

4

Release the stretch briefly. Do the stretch 2 times with each arm.

Shoulder Stretch—across the Body

Stand with proper posture. Bring one arm across your body, resting your hand on your shoulder.

1

Using your other hand, gently pull your elbow farther across your body.

2

Feel the stretch along the back of your shoulder.

3

Hold for 20 seconds.

4

Release the stretch briefly. Do the stretch 2 times with each arm.

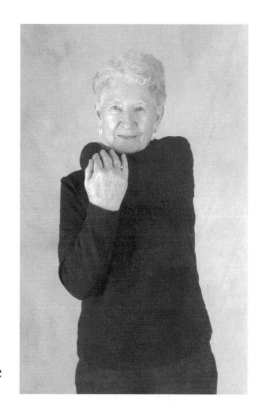

Chest Stretch

Stand with proper posture and clasp your hands behind your back.

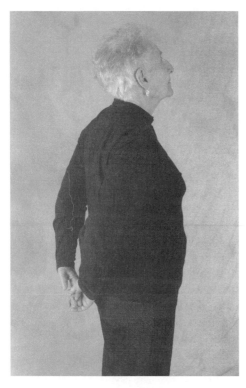

1

Gently pull your shoulder blades down and together, lifting up through your chest.

2

Feel this stretch along the front of your shoulders and chest.

3

Hold for 20 seconds.

4

Release the stretch briefly. Repeat.

Calf Stretch

Stand with your hands on the edge of the pool. Place one foot behind your body with both knees bent. Maintain proper posture throughout the exercise.

1

With your toes pointing straight ahead and your heels flat on the floor, gently lunge forward.

2

Feel the stretch in your calf.

3

Hold for 20 seconds.

4

Release the stretch briefly. Do the stretch 2 times with each leg.

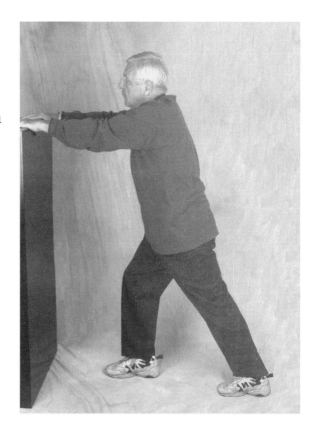

Hamstring Stretch

Stand with proper posture. Set one foot on the wall of the pool at about knee height.

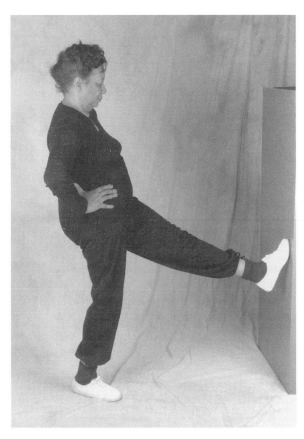

1
Keeping your back straight, lean forward at your waist, being careful not to stretch too far and lose proper form.

2
Feel the gentle stretch along the back of your thigh.

3
Hold for 20 seconds.

4
Release the stretch briefly. Do the stretch 2 times with each leg.

Thigh Stretch

Stand with proper posture and place one hand on the edge of the pool.

1

Grasp one foot and bring the heel to your buttocks; do not bend at the waist.

2

Feel the stretch along the front of your thigh.

3

Hold for 20 seconds.

4

Release the stretch briefly. Do the stretch 2 times with each leg.

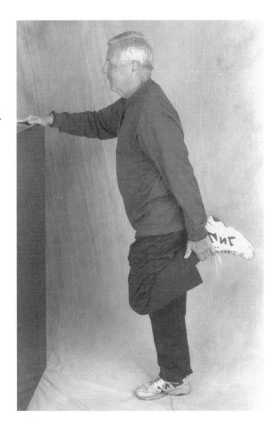

CONCLUSION

This pool program provides another strength-training option for older adults. You may use the program regularly, or you might try it as an occasional change from your usual strength-training program. Either way, you should find the pool a comfortable place for exercise.

Lorie A. Schleck is a physical therapist at Fairview Rehabilitation Services. She received her BS degree in physical therapy from the University of Minnesota and her MA degree in counseling psychology from St. Mary's University of Minnesota. Lorie and her husband, Jim, have a son, Ben, and a daughter, Kara.

9

Strength Training in a Chair

Julie Varno, MS, PT
Lorie A. Schleck, MA, PT

This program takes 20 to 30 minutes.

Do it 2 to 3 times a week.

A 48-hour break is recommended between each session.

EQUIPMENT NEEDED:
    Comfortable, heavy chair with armrests
    Chair or stool
    Length of resistance band (3 to 4 feet)
    Loop of resistance band
    Towel or belt
    Firm pillow

For many of us, it is unsafe—if not impossible—to exercise while standing up. An arthritic hip, an injured knee, or other medical problems could make standing painful and difficult. Balance problems, which are also common with advancing age, can make standing exercises unsteady or unsafe. In both cases, seated exercises are a good alternative.

If we are recovering from a prolonged illness or hospital stay, a seated strength-training program is a first step to regaining our strength. As our strength improves, we can progress to a program involving standing exercises.

Those of us who are confined to a wheelchair draw particular benefits from strength training. Whether or not we require assistance, transferring from a wheelchair to a bed or car is safer and smoother when important muscle groups are strong. Furthermore, regular stretching exercises help prevent slouching, which often occurs after long periods in a wheelchair.

TIPS FOR STRENGTH TRAINING IN A CHAIR

The exercises in this program are not only safe, but when performed correctly, they're as effective as the other exercises in this book.

Adapt this program to your own needs and abilities. For example, if you have use of only one arm or leg, exercise only that side. If you do not have use of your legs, focus on the arm exercises. If certain exercises are easy, do more repetitions. If some exercises are hard, do fewer repetitions.

You should never be exhausted during or after exercise. If this happens, stop immediately. And, although your breathing should be faster than it is when you're at rest, you should never be short of breath. If you are, stop immediately.

THE PROGRAM

For many people, Strength Training in a Chair is a transitional program. If you are able, use this program until you are strong enough to switch to one of the standing programs in this book.

These exercises require proper posture. Sit tall with your head up and your ears aligned with your shoulders. Your feet should rest comfortably but firmly on the floor.

Strength Training in a Chair consists of a warm-up session, strengthening exercises, and warm-down stretching exercises. You may want to meet with a physical therapist or other health-care professional before beginning this program. A trained professional can help make sure you are exercising properly.

Exercise Guidelines
- Wear comfortable, nonbinding clothing.
- Maintain proper body alignment: Sit up tall with your feet firmly on the floor.
- Perform each exercise slowly and smoothly.
- Do each exercise in a pain-free range of motion.
- Do not increase resistance too quickly.
- Begin with a warm-up session.
- End with the warm-down stretching exercises.

Safety Reminders
- Do not hold your breath while exercising.
- Stop immediately if you are short of breath.
- Stop immediately if you become fatigued.
- Exercises should not cause pain.

WARM-UP EXERCISES

The purpose of the warm-up is to increase blood flow to key muscle groups just before strength training. The warm-up takes four to five minutes. It will get your heart pumping a little harder and the blood moving a little faster to prepare your muscles for the work ahead.

If you cannot do some of the warm-up exercises, simply increase the amount of time you spend on the others, so your total warm-up lasts four minutes.

The warm-up should not leave you tired or short of breath. If it does, decrease the amount of time you spend on each exercise until your warm-up lasts only two or three minutes.

Ankle Circles

Sit with proper posture. Lift one foot off the ground, leaving a slight bend at the knee.

1

Slowly move your foot in a circle, clockwise, 10 times.

2

Switch directions. Slowly move your foot in a circle, counterclockwise, 10 times. Repeat with your other foot.

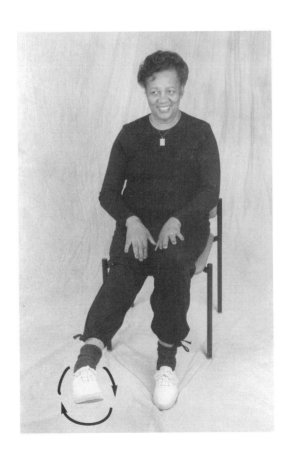

Toe and Heel Taps

Sit with proper posture.

1

Lift your heels and touch your toes to the ground.

2

Lift your toes and touch your heels to the ground.

3

Continue alternating toes to heels for 1 to 1 ½ minutes.

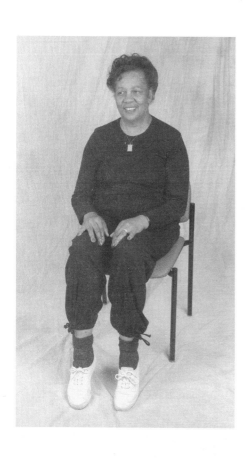 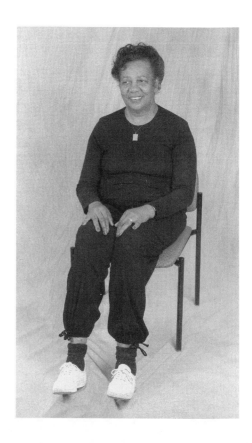

Marching

Sit with proper posture.

1

Lift one knee so your foot is just slightly off the ground.

2

Return that foot to the ground while lifting the other knee.

3

Continue for 1 to 1 ½ minutes.

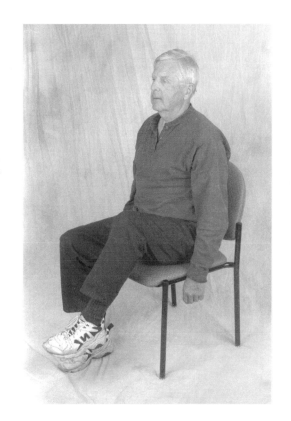

Arm Circles

Sit with proper posture. Bring your arms out to the sides, slightly below shoulder level.

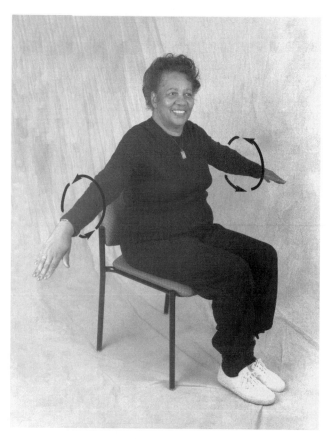

1

Make small, backward circles with your arms for 30 seconds.

2

Make small, forward circles with your arms for 30 seconds.

3

If 30 seconds is too long, do as many circles as you can without getting tired.

This completes your warm-up. You are now ready to start the strength-training exercises.

STRENGTHENING EXERCISES

The strengthening portion of this program consists of ten exercises for key muscle groups in your arms, legs, and trunk. If an exercise causes pain, limit your range of motion during that exercise. For example, if it hurts to straighten your leg, don't straighten it all the way. If you still have pain while limiting the motion, do not do the exercise.

Some exercises call for a length of resistance band. Others call for a loop of band. To make a loop, tie the ends of the band together. You might want to try the exercises without a band at first, adding it when your strength improves. You may need help adjusting the band for certain exercises.

For exercises without a Thera-Band resistance band:
- Begin with 10 repetitions.
- As the exercises get easier, progress to 12 and then to 15 repetitions.
- Next, progress to two sets of 10, then 12, then 15 repetitions.
- Finally, if able, progress to three sets of 10, then 12, then 15 repetitions.

For exercises with a Thera-Band resistance band:
- Begin with 10 repetitions.
- As the exercises get easier, progress to 12 and then to 15 repetitions.
- Next, move to a higher level band and do 10, then 12, then 15 repetitions.
- After you reach your ideal level of resistance, do two sets of 10, then 12, then 15.
- Finally, if able, progress to three sets of 10, then 12, then 15 repetitions.

Arm Curls
(use a length of resistance band)

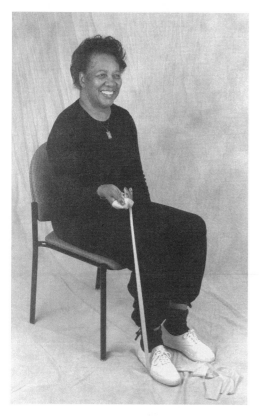

Sit with proper posture. Step on one end of the band (or tie the band to the leg of the chair). Grasp the other end in one hand, palm up.

1

Keep your upper body still and your elbow close to your body. Bend your arm and bring your hand to your shoulder. (Do not bend your wrist.)

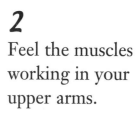

2
Feel the muscles working in your upper arms.

3
Return to the starting position. Repeat 10 times with each arm.

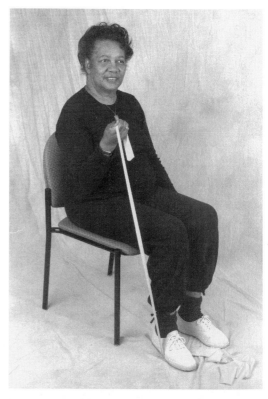

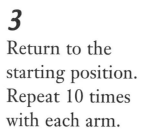

Push-Ups
(use a chair with armrests)

Sit with proper posture, placing both hands on the armrests directly beneath your shoulders. Keep your feet firmly on the floor throughout the exercise.

1

Gently push yourself up off the chair, lifting your buttocks a few inches off the seat. Do not lock your elbows.

2

Feel the muscles working in your upper arms.

3

Slowly lower yourself back down to the starting position. Repeat 10 times.

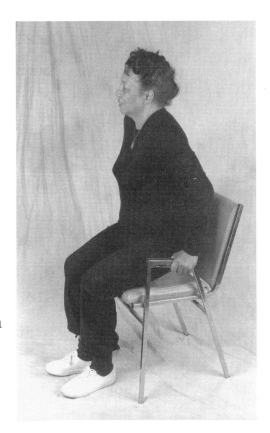

This is a fairly difficult exercise. If you cannot lift yourself, you can still benefit from trying.

Shoulder Blade Squeeze
(use a length of resistance band)

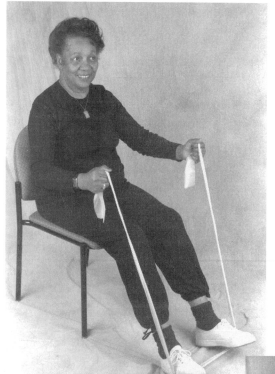

Sit with proper posture. Extend both legs, keeping your heels on the floor. Hook the band around both feet, grasping one end in each hand.

1

Squeeze your shoulder blades together while pulling your arms back, leading with your elbows. Feel the muscles working in your shoulders and upper back.

2

Return to the starting position. Repeat 10 times.

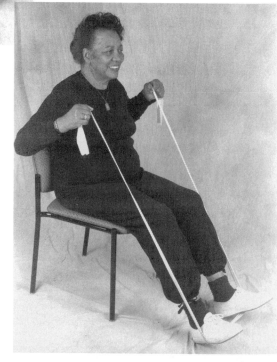

Heel Lifts

Sit with proper posture. Place both feet on the floor, about shoulder-width apart.

1

Slowly lift both heels off the floor.

2

Feel the muscles working in your calves.

3

Slowly lower your heels back to the floor. Repeat 10 times.

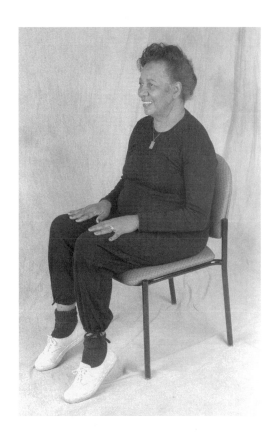

When this exercise gets too easy, go on to the next exercise—toe points.

Toe Points
(use a length of resistance band)

Do this exercise only after heel lifts become too easy.

Sit with proper posture. Extend one leg, keeping the heel on the floor. Flex your foot and hook the band around the ball of the foot. Grasp the band in your hands and pull it taut.

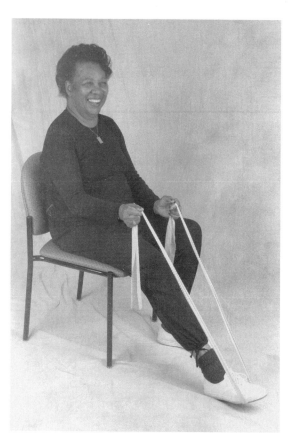

1

Slowly point your toes against the band's resistance.

2

Feel the muscles working in your calf.

3

Slowly return to the starting position. Repeat 10 times with each foot.

Lower Leg "Kicks"

Sit with proper posture.

1

Flexing your toes, extend one leg until it is straight.

2

Feel the muscles working along the top of your thigh.

3

Slowly return to the starting position. Repeat 10 times with each leg.

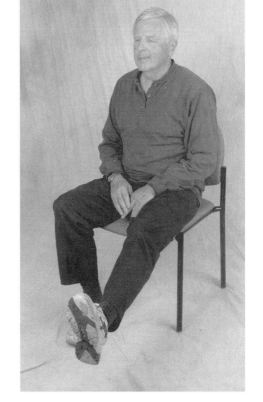

If this exercise is too easy, do two or three sets. If it is still too easy, go on to the next exercise—lower leg "kicks" using a Thera-Band resistance band.

Lower Leg "Kicks"–with a Band
(use a loop of resistance band)

Do this exercise only after lower leg "kicks" become too easy.

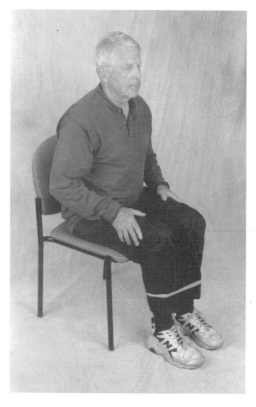

Sit with proper posture. Loop a band around your ankles.

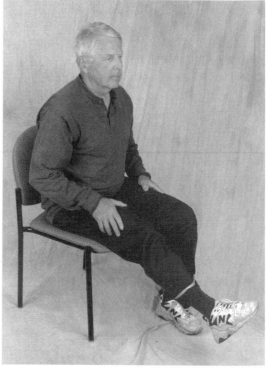

1
Flexing your toes,
extend one leg until it is straight.

2
Feel the muscles working along the top of your thigh.

3
Slowly return to the starting position. Repeat 10
times with each leg.

Heel Drags

Sit with proper posture.

1

Place one heel on the ground, as far in front of you as you can.

2

Drag the heel along the floor until your foot sits flat.

3

To create more resistance, push your heel into the ground as you drag it toward your chair.
Repeat 10 times with each foot.

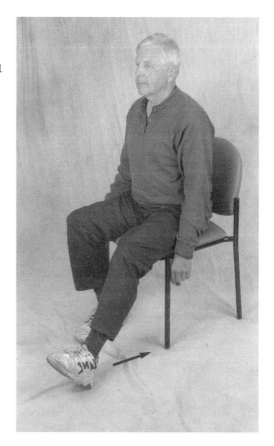

Pillow Squeeze
(use a firm pillow)

Sit with proper posture and place the pillow between your knees.

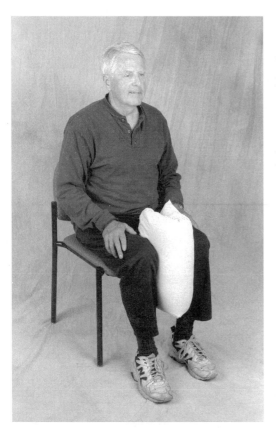

1

Squeeze your knees together for 5 seconds.

2

Relax. Repeat 10 times.

Knee Push
(use a loop of resistance band)

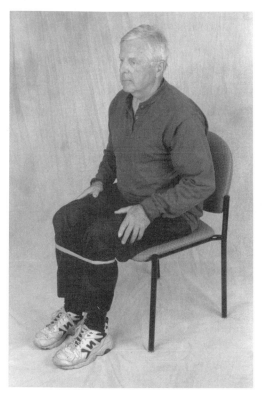

Sit with proper
posture, your feet
shoulder-width
apart. Loop the band
around your legs,
just below the knees.

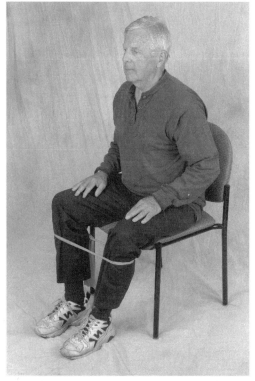

1
Push your knees out to the sides
against the band's resistance.

2
Relax and return to the starting
position. Repeat 10 times.

This completes your strengthening exercises. You are now
ready to "warm down" with some stretching exercises.

WARM-DOWN STRETCHING EXERCISES

A gentle stretching session is the perfect way to "warm down." Stretching also makes your joints and muscles more flexible. In fact, stretching has been shown to decrease many aches and pains associated with advancing age.

Ease into each stretch until you feel a gentle pull or tug along the muscle. Do not bounce. You should not feel pain. If you do, review the technique for the stretch and try again. If you still have pain, leave that particular stretch out of your routine.

Do all stretches while sitting tall and straight, your ears aligned with your shoulders.

Nose-to-Shoulder Stretch

Sit with proper posture.

1

Turn your head so your nose is over
your shoulder.

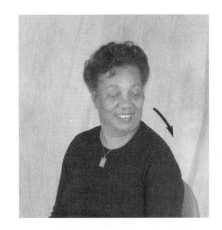

2

Bring your head down, moving your
nose toward your shoulder.

3

Hold for 20 seconds, feeling the stretch in your neck.

4

Bring your head up.

5

Return to the starting position. Do this stretch 2
times on each side.

Shoulder Stretch—across the Body

Sit with proper posture. Bring one arm across your body so your hand is near the opposite shoulder.

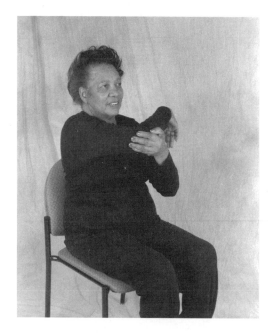

1

Using your other hand, gently pull your elbow farther across your body.

2

Feel the stretch along the back of your shoulder.

3

Hold for 20 seconds.

4

Release the stretch briefly. Do this stretch 2 times with each arm.

Shoulder Stretch—over the Head

Sit with proper posture. Place one hand toward the back of your neck, pointing your elbow in the air.

1

Using your other hand, gently pull your elbow toward the middle of your back.

2

Feel the stretch along your shoulder.

3

Hold for 20 seconds.

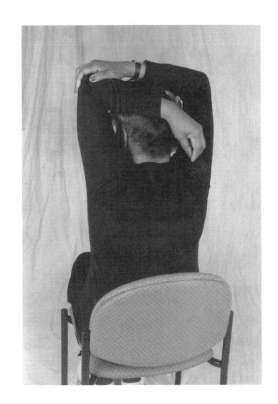

4

Release the stretch briefly. Do this stretch 2 times with each arm.

Chest Stretch

Sit with proper posture.

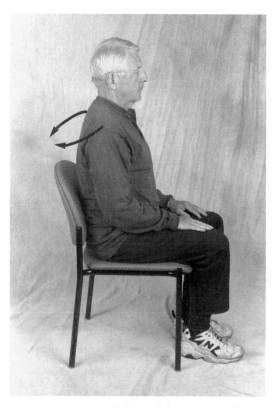

1

Lifting up through your chest, gently pull your shoulders back, bringing your shoulder blades together and down.

2

Feel this stretch along the front of your shoulders and chest.

3

Hold for 5 seconds.

4

Release the stretch briefly. Repeat 10 times.

Calf Stretch
(use a belt or towel)

Sit with proper posture. Loop the belt or towel around the toes of one foot, keeping the heel of that foot on the ground. Grasp the ends in both hands.

1

Use the belt or towel to bend your foot back toward your knee.

2

Feel the stretch in your calf.

3

Hold for 20 seconds.

4

Release the stretch briefly. Do the stretch 2 times with each leg.

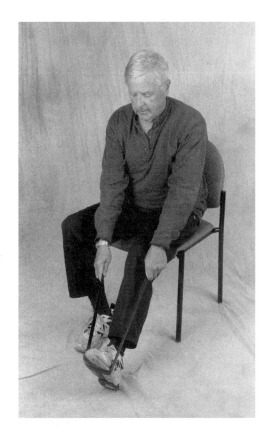

Hamstring and Calf Stretch

Sit with proper posture. Set one foot on the seat of a chair or stool.

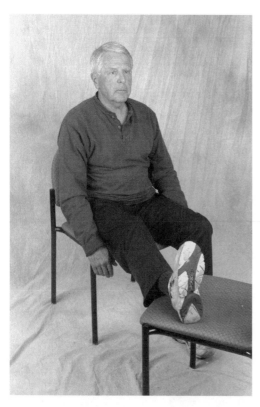

1
Flex your toes.

2
Feel the stretch along the back of your thigh and calf.

3
Hold for 20 seconds.

4
Release the stretch briefly. Do the stretch 2 times with each leg.

When this exercise gets too easy, go on to the next exercise— hamstring and calf stretch using a towel.

Hamstring and Calf Stretch— with a Towel

Do this exercise only after the hamstring and calf stretch becomes too easy.

Sit with proper posture. Set one foot on the seat of a chair or stool. Loop the towel around the ball of your foot and grasp it in both hands.

1

Flex your toes. (Do not bend forward at the waist.)

2

Feel the stretch along the back of your thigh and calf.

3

Hold for 20 seconds.

4

Release the stretch briefly. Do the stretch 2 times with each leg.

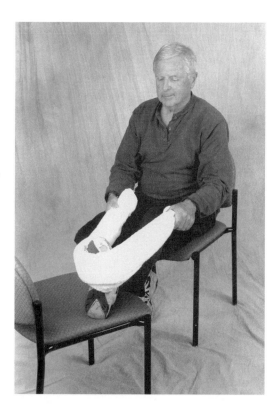

CONCLUSION

When standing exercises are unsafe, painful, or impossible, a seated strength-training program will help you build the strong, flexible muscles you need. If you are recovering from a long illness, use this program until you are able to progress to standing exercises.

Julie Varno is a physical therapist at Fairview Rehabilitation Services. She received her BS degree from Winona State University in Winona, Minnesota, and her MS in physical therapy from the University of Alabama at Birmingham. She has a special interest in neurological and vestibular disorders. Julie and her husband, Tom, have one daughter, Melissa, and one son, Jeremy.

Lorie A. Schleck is a physical therapist at Fairview Rehabilitation Services. She received her BS degree in physical therapy from the University of Minnesota and her MA degree in counseling psychology from St. Mary's University of Minnesota. Lorie and her husband, Jim, have a son, Ben, and a daughter, Kara.

10

Strength Training in Bed

Debbie Hanka, PT
Lorie A. Schleck, MA, PT

This program takes about 15 minutes.
Do it every day.

EQUIPMENT NEEDED:
    Bed with a firm mattress
    Length of resistance band (3 or 4 foot)
    Loop of resistance band
    Towel or belt
    Pillow (optional)

Sometimes it's difficult to exercise while standing or sitting. We might feel weak, dizzy, or off-balance. Perhaps we're restricted to a bed because of illness or injury. At times like these, strength training in bed can help us maintain or regain our strength and flexibility. There is little risk of falling, and the bed offers plenty of support. Plus, the exercises in this program are very gentle, so there's no need to worry about overdoing it.

PRECAUTIONS

In addition to the precautions listed in chapter 2, you should consider the following before you begin strength training:

• **If you have had a hip replacement, do not use this program.** The exercises required after hip replacement surgery are different from the exercises described here. Follow the precautions outlined by your surgeon or physical therapist.

• **If you have recently had a serious illness, talk with your doctor before starting a strength-training program.** Every illness is different. Your doctor can tell you which exercises are appropriate for your condition, and which are not.

• **If you have heart disease, consult your doctor.** Depending on your condition, certain exercises may cause dangerous symptoms.

THE PROGRAM

Strength Training in Bed consists of a warm-up session, strengthening exercises, and warm-down stretching exercises. You may want to meet with a physical therapist or other health-care professional before beginning this program. A trained professional can help make sure you are exercising properly.

Many people find that exercising in bed first thing in the morning helps loosen up their joints so they can start the day. If you use this program to alleviate morning stiffness, do one set of 10 repetitions every morning. But remember, the body gets specific benefits from exercising in a sitting or standing position. If you are able, use a second strength-training program two or three times a week. See the guide in chapter 2 to determine which program is right for you.

If you are recovering from an illness or injury, these bed exercises will help you regain your strength. But for most people they're not enough. When and if you are able, you should progress to Strength Training in a Chair, and then to an appropriate program with standing exercises.

If you are unable to leave your bed for medical or safety reasons, continue strength training every day. Regular exercise will help you maintain the strength and flexibility you need to stay active and enjoy a greater amount of independence.

For maximum safety, always move to the center of the bed while exercising.

Exercise Guidelines
- Wear comfortable, nonbinding clothing.
- Maintain proper body alignment.
- Perform each exercise slowly and smoothly.
- Do each exercise in a pain-free range of motion.
- Do not increase resistance too quickly.
- Begin with a warm-up session.
- End with the warm-down stretching exercises.

Safety Reminders
- Discuss any precautions with your physician or physical therapist.
- Always exercise in the center of the bed.
- Do not hold your breath while exercising.
- Stop immediately if you are short of breath.
- Stop immediately if you become fatigued.
- Exercises should not cause pain.

WARM-UP EXERCISES

This warm-up consists of a sequence of isometric exercises. In an isometric exercise, a muscle contracts but the body doesn't move. Pushing your arm into the bed, for example, is an isometric exercise.

Isometric exercises will increase blood flow to your muscles, preparing them for strength training. Begin by lying on your back with your arms at your side, hands flat with palms down. If you are comfortable without a pillow beneath your head, remove the pillow and lie with your head on the mattress.

You will push specific parts of your body down into the bed, holding each successive contraction until you release them all at the end of the sequence. Move immediately from one contraction to the next. With practice, it will take only one or two seconds to complete one contraction and move on to the next. The entire isometric sequence should take about ten seconds.

Warm-up Sequence

Lie flat on your back, palms down.

1

Push each body part into the bed in the following order (hold each contraction as you add the next):

     a. Back of your head

     b. Back of both shoulders

     c. Palms of both hands

     d. Both hips

     e. Back of both knees

     f. Both heels

2
Release them all at once.

3
Relax. Repeat 3 to 5 times.

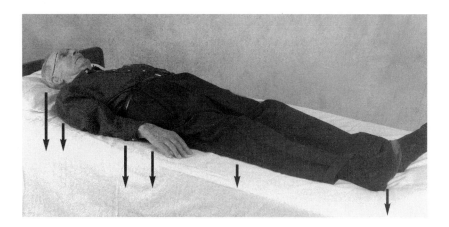

This completes your warm-up. You are now ready to start the strength-training exercises.

STRENGTHENING EXERCISES

The strengthening portion of this program includes eight exercises for key muscle groups in your arms, legs, and trunk. If an exercise causes pain, limit your range of motion during that exercise. For example, if it hurts to straighten your leg, don't straighten it all the way. If you still have pain while limiting the motion, do not do the exercise.

Some exercises call for a length of resistance band. Others call for a loop of band. To make a loop, tie the ends of the band together. You may want to exercise without a band at first, adding it only when you feel ready.

For exercises without a Thera-Band resistance band:
- Unless directed otherwise, begin with 10 repetitions.
- As the exercises get easier, progress to 12 and then to 15 repetitions.
- Next, progress to two sets of 10, then 12, then 15 repetitions.
- Finally, if able, progress to three sets of 10, then 12, then 15 repetitions.

For exercises with a Thera-Band resistance band:
- Begin with 10 repetitions.
- As the exercises get easier, progress to 12 and then to 15 repetitions.
- Next, move to a higher level band and do 10, then 12, then 15 repetitions.
- After you reach your ideal level of resistance, do two sets of 10, then 12, then 15.
- Finally, if able, progress to three sets of 10, then 12, then 15 repetitions.

NOTE: This is not a complete strength-training program. It is impossible to work all the muscles while exercising in bed. However, this is a good starting point if you are weak from illness or inactivity. It is also an excellent program to use if you like to exercise before getting out of bed. For those who are restricted to their bed and who do not expect to progress to chair exercises, this program is essential for maintaining strength.

Ankle Pumps

Lie flat on your back. Perform this exercise smoothly and slowly without pause.

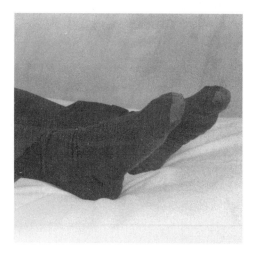

1

Point your toes toward the foot of the bed.

2

Switch directions, flexing your foot toward the head of the bed.

3

Feel the muscles working in your calves and shins. Repeat 20 times.

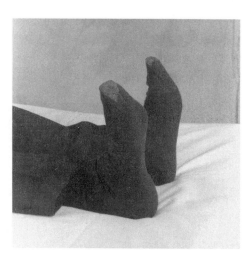

If you are able, rest for 60 seconds, then do another set of 20 repetitions.

Heel Slides

Lie flat on your back, palms down.

1
Slowly bend one knee, sliding your heel along the bed toward your buttocks.

2
Pause for 1 or 2 seconds, then slide your heel back, straightening your leg.

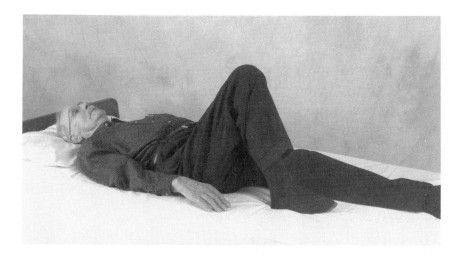

3
Feel the muscles working in your thigh and hip. Repeat 10 times with each leg.

Buttocks Squeeze

Lie flat on your back with your knees bent.

1

Tighten your buttocks by squeezing your "cheeks" together. (Put your hands on your buttocks to feel the muscles tighten.)

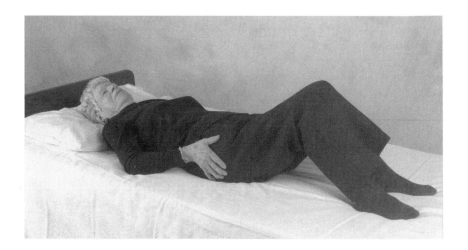

2

Hold for 5 seconds.

3

Relax briefly. Repeat 10 times.

When this exercise gets too easy, go on to the next exercise—bridging.

Bridging

Do this exercise only after the buttocks squeeze becomes too easy.

Lie flat on your back with your knees bent.

1

Tighten your buttocks by squeezing your "cheeks" together.

2

Slowly lift your hips 2 to 3 inches off the bed. Feel the muscles working in your buttocks and thighs.

3

Slowly lower your hips back to the bed.

4

Relax. Repeat 10 times.

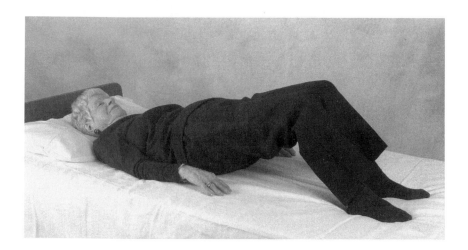

Leg Slides

Lie flat on your back with your feet together, toes pointed toward the ceiling.

1

Slide one leg out to the side. (Do not allow your leg to bend.)

2

Feel the muscles working in your thigh.

3

Slowly slide your leg back to the starting position. Repeat 10 times with each leg.

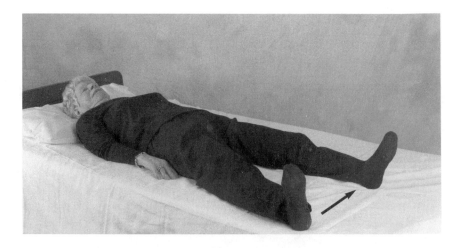

When this exercise gets too easy, go on to the next exercise— side leg lifts.

Side Leg Lifts

Lie on your side, using a pillow or your forearm to support your head and neck. Line your feet up with your body, being careful not to bend at the waist. Bend your bottom leg—the one resting on the bed—to add support and stability.

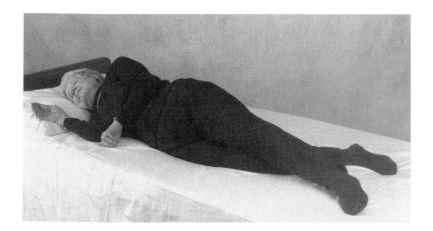

1
Keeping your top leg straight, slowly lift it about 12 inches off the bed.

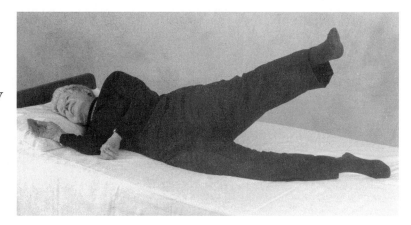

2
Feel the muscles working in your hip and thigh.

3
Slowly return to the starting position. Repeat 10 times with each leg.

Arm Lifts

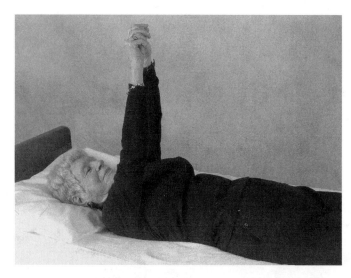

Lie flat on your back. Reach both hands above your chest, keeping your arms straight.

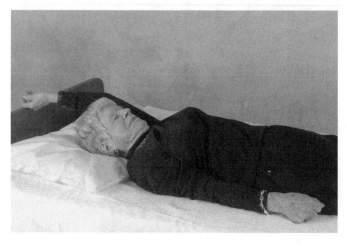

1
Bring one arm over-head and the other down to your hip.

2
Switch directions, bringing the opposite arm overhead and the other to your hip.

3
Feel the muscles working in your shoulders and upper arms. Repeat 10 times.

When this exercise gets too easy, go on to the next exercise— arm lifts using a Thera-Band resistance band.

Arm Lifts—with a Band
(use a length of resistance band)

Do this exercise only after the arm lifts become too easy.

Lie flat on your back.
Reach both hands above
your chest, keeping your
arms straight. Grasp the
band with your hands about
18 to 24 inches apart.

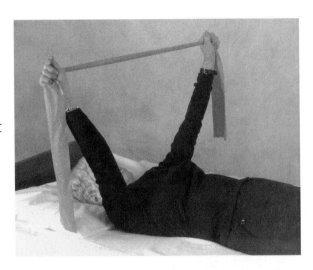

1

Bring one arm overhead
and the other toward your
hip, stretching the band as
you do so.

2

Switch directions, bringing
your opposite arm over-
head and the other arm
toward your hip.

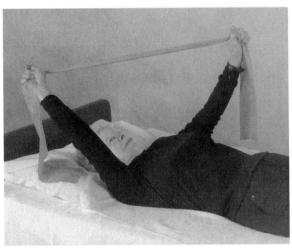

3

Feel the muscles working
in your upper arms. Repeat 10 times.

If this exercise is too difficult, move your hands farther apart
on the band.

   This completes your strengthening exercises. You are now
ready to "warm down" with some stretching exercises.

WARM-DOWN STRETCHING EXERCISES

A gentle stretching session is the perfect way to "warm down." Stretching also makes your joints and muscles more flexible. In fact, stretching has been shown to decrease many aches and pains associated with advancing age.

Ease into each stretch until you feel a gentle pull or tug along the muscle. Do not bounce. You should not feel pain. If you do, review the technique for the stretch and try again. If you still have pain, leave that particular stretch out of your routine. Perform each stretch twice, holding for twenty seconds.

Ankle Stretch
(use a belt or towel)

Standing and walking require flexible calf muscles and good ankle motion. This exercise helps with both. Lying in bed for extended periods makes the calf muscles prone to tightness, so this exercise is particularly important if you are recovering from an illness.

Sit up with both legs extended in front of you. Hook the belt or towel over the balls of your feet, holding one end in each hand.

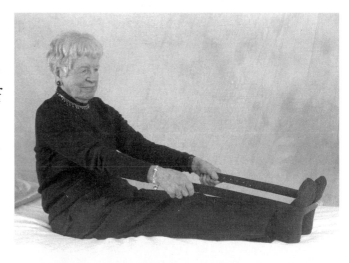

1
Gently pull the belt or towel, bending your feet toward your body.

2
Feel the stretch in your calves.

3
Hold for 20 seconds.

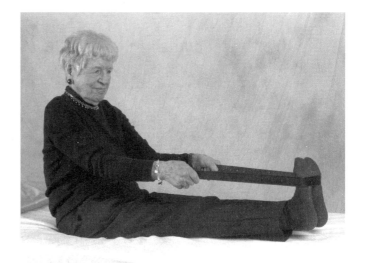

4
Release the stretch briefly. Repeat.

Hamstring Stretch

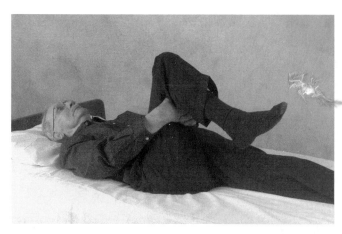

Lie flat on your back and pull one knee toward your chest. Your knee should be over your hip and your thigh should be perpendicular to the bed. Grasp your thigh with both hands.

1
Straighten your leg.

2
Feel the gentle stretch along the back of your thigh.

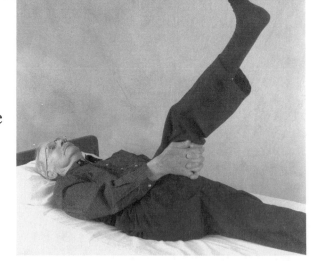

3
Hold for 20 seconds.

4
Release the stretch briefly. Do this stretch 2 times with each leg.

Hip Stretch

Lie flat on your stomach.

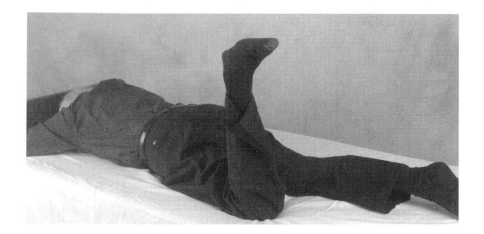

1

Bend one knee, bringing your heel toward
your buttocks.

2

Feel the gentle stretch along the front of your thigh.

3

Hold for 20 seconds.

4

Release the stretch briefly. Do this stretch 2 times
with each leg.

"Butterfly" Stretch

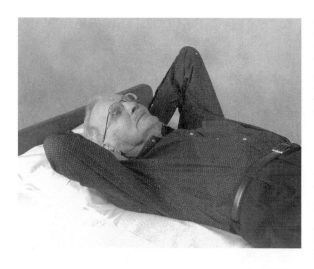

Lie flat on your back.
Interlace your fingers and
place your hands behind
your head.

1

Pull your elbows toward
the bed. (Be careful not to
pull on your neck during
this stretch.)

2

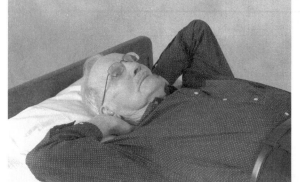

Feel the stretch along the
front of your shoulders
and chest.

3

Hold for 20 seconds.

4

Release the stretch briefly.
Repeat.

CONCLUSION

Exercising in bed may be an important part of your normal "get up and go" routine. Or, perhaps you're using it to transition from illness to health, from weakness to strength. Maybe you're restricted to your bed and simply want to maintain the strength you have. Regardless, this program is an excellent opportunity to make strength training a regular part of your life.

Debbie Hanka is the program coordinator for Preventing Falls in Older Adults at Fairview Ridges Hospital. She received her BS degree in physical therapy from the University of Minnesota. Debbie and her husband, Greg, have three children, Emily, Ben, and Ian.

Lorie A. Schleck is a physical therapist at Fairview Rehabilitation Services. She received her BS degree in physical therapy from the University of Minnesota and her MA degree in counseling psychology from St. Mary's University of Minnesota. Lorie and her husband, Jim, have a son, Ben, and a daughter, Kara.

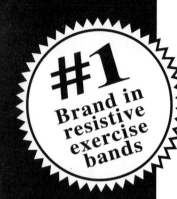